Wendy Leebov's

# Essentials for Great
# Patient Experiences

Wendy Leebov's

# *Essentials for Great Patient Experiences*

## No-Nonsense Solutions with Gratifying Results

Wendy Leebov, Ed.D.

Health Forum, Inc.
An American Hospital Association Company
CHICAGO

AHA
press

Printed in the United States of America—04/08

Cover design by Cheri Kusek

ISBN: 978-1-55648-352-3

Item Number: 042202

**Library of Congress Cataloging-in-Publication Data**

Leebov, Wendy.
   Wendy Leebov's essentials for great patient experiences : no-nonsense solutions with gratifying results / Wendy Leebov.
       p. ; cm.
   "Includes a collection of . . . articles published originally . . . in Hospitals and Health Networks Online"—Pref.
   Includes bibliographical references and index.
   ISBN 978-1-55648-352-3 (alk. paper)
   1. Patient satisfaction. 2. Medical personnel and patient. I. American Hospital Association. II. Hospitals & health networks (Online) III. Title. IV. Title: Essentials for great patient experiences.
   [DNLM: 1. Hospital-Patient Relations—Collected Works. 2. Quality Assurance, Health Care—methods—Collected Works. 3. Health Services Administration—Collected Works. 4. Patient Acceptance of Health Care—Collected Works. 5. Patient Satisfaction—Collected Works. 6. Professional-Patient Relations—Collected Works. WX 153 L482w 2008]
   R727.3.L353 2008
   610.69'6—dc22
                    2007051909

*I dedicate this book to my wonderful sister,*
Linda Leebov Goldston

Linda's life-changing experiences as a patient at every level of our health care system have filled me with gratitude for the throngs of people in health care who perform miracles, every day and night, with remarkable expertise and compassion. Linda's experiences have also sparked in me new insights about the compelling challenges we must embrace to create even more healing environments, and healing inter-actions, for patients and families who depend on us during times of personal trauma, fragility, and need.

# Contents

# List of Figures and Tools

# About the Author

**Wendy Leebov, Ed.D.,** is a passionate advocate for creating healing environments for patients, families, and the entire health care team. She has twenty-five years of experience in helping leaders lead effectively and launch and sustain far-reaching strategies that enhance the patient and employee experience.

During two decades of service with the Albert Einstein Healthcare Network in Philadelphia, Wendy most recently held the position of vice president, human resources. She also founded the Einstein Consulting Group, a firm respected for helping more than 300 health care organizations with strategies to achieve care with compassion and leadership effectiveness.

Now an independent consultant on leadership development, the patient experience, and organizational change, Wendy is also a compelling presenter of keynote presentations and designer and facilitator of workshops and learning processes.

Wendy received her bachelor of arts degree in sociology/anthropology from Oberlin College. She earned her master's in education and doctorate in human development from the Harvard Graduate School of Education.

In addition to writing "The Executive Tool Kit" column for *Hospitals and Health Networks OnLine,* Wendy Leebov has written more than ten books for health care leaders, including *The Indispensable Health Care Manager: Success Strategies for a Changing Environment* (with G. Scott), *Health Care Managers in Transition: Shifting Roles for Changing Organizations* (also with G. Scott), *Achieving Impressive Customer Service: Strategies for the Health Care Manager* (with G. Scott and L. Olson), and *Service Quality Improvement: The Customer Satisfaction Strategy for Health Care* (with G. Scott).

# Preface

It's time to lead our teams beyond customer service to meet the challenge of creating the *great* patient experience.

It's time to create even more healing environments, where vulnerable people can come to us for excellent medical care, compassion, and support.

It's time to embrace *care with compassion* as our goal and build the culture, processes, communication, continuity, and teamwork that deliver on that promise.

This book is a collection of mind-stretching articles, published originally as part of "The Executive Tool Kit" feature in *Hospitals and Health Networks OnLine.* In addition to the articles, you'll find many practical tools never before published—tools that help you to implement the suggested strategies with speed and ease.

At the end of this book, you'll find an appendix containing "Additional Resources for Health Care Leaders." This section refers you to books, articles, and other sources, all to help you delve deeper into topics of particular interest.

Giving patients great experiences must be our goal in every health care setting. Here's hoping these tools will help you to *be* more effective and also to *feel* more gratified as you care for your patients.

*Wendy Leebov, Ed.D.*
*Philadelphia*

Wendy Leebov's

*Essentials for Great*

*Patient Experiences*

# Chapter 1

• • •

# Empathy Fitness
# for Leaders

*Take time to learn how patients experience
your care and service.*

At a leadership meeting, try an experiment. Ask people to suggest
how a caregiver should respond to this outcry from a patient:

"I'm in terrible pain. I need more medicine now!"

My prediction is that most will suggest task-oriented or information-
gathering approaches—responses that move immediately toward fix-
ing the problem. For instance:

- "What hurts?"
- "Did this just start?"
- "How would you rate your pain from 1 to 10?"
- "Let me look at your chart and see when you can have more
  medicine."
- "I'll call the doctor and see if there's something else you could
  have for the pain."

No doubt, leaders' quickness to get more information and act
on the problem comes from their caring. The problem is that the
patient's outcry is fraught with feeling, and responses from the *head,*
not the *heart,* ignore this feeling. Responses from the head convey no
empathy. The result: the patient experiences the caregiver as insensi-
tive or impersonal, even if that caregiver tries to find a way to provide pain relief.

Many caring caregivers rarely express empathy yet feel surprised when patients report their care as competent but perfunctory and impersonal—reflective of a factory, not a healing environment.

A one-sentence acknowledgment of the feeling—an expression from the caregiver's heart—would do wonders in showing the staff member's caring. The caregiver can say, "I'm so sorry you're in pain" or "I want to help you!" and then proceed to fix the problem.

## It Starts at the Top

In health care these days, task orientation is epidemic. Many leaders appear detached from the emotional aspects of the patient's experience. They are busy, busy, busy—solving problems, handling crises, controlling cost, pursuing goals, going to meetings, ironing out snags, building the business, handling complaints, getting things done, and much more. They expect their teams to be highly productive and hardworking, too.

This is a concern: We talk about creating great experiences for patients, but how can we possibly do that if we don't see the patients' experience through their eyes and demonstrate empathy for their experience in our words, actions, and decisions?

The decisions leaders are making need to be informed not only by savvy planning but also by emotional intelligence about the patient's experience. This will enable leaders to devise and support optimal patient experiences and guide their teams in connecting to patients and families with heartfelt sensitivity.

## Empathy Fitness Exercises

It takes deliberate effort to stay tuned in to the emotional aspects of the patient experience. It takes an empathy fitness program. While leadership rounding is wonderful, many leaders approach it with a focus on identifying and solving problems, rather than understanding the patient experience through the patients' eyes.

Leaders should engage in one exercise a month. Spread the learning by spending fifteen minutes of monthly leader meetings focusing on stories and insights about the patients' experience, *not* on solutions and improvements.

## Empathy Fitness Exercises: Some Examples

**Do a walk-through:**
- With a colleague, undergo a service—one of you as a patient, the other as a companion. Look. Listen. Feel. Resist thinking about fixes.
- Tell staff what you're doing. You are not hunting for problems or watching their performance. Instead, you want to see services through the eyes of the patient. Ask them to treat you as they normally would treat a patient or a family member.
- Walk through the whole experience.
  - —Start with setting up an appointment. Begin your experience at the parking lot or other transportation point and end by returning there. Pretend that you have never been to this service before. Get directions. Ask any questions you might have if you were a patient and family member.
  - —When you arrive, tell the front-desk staff that you want to experience the service, so you're going through it as if the two of you were a real patient and family member. Ask them to check you in as they would any other patient and family member. Fill out the forms. Wait your turn. Pay your co-payment if they ask. And so on.
  - —When you're in the exam room, undress if the patient would. Wait as the patient would. If the patient would do a peak flow meter, you do it, too. Experience every part that you can without risk to yourself.
- As you proceed, look through the lens of a patient or family member. See things as they would. Hear as they would. Try to think and feel as they would.
- Afterward, jot down notes about your feelings, anxieties, and satisfactions. Have your colleague do the same. Don't solve problems and identify improvements. Focus on the details of the experience from your view as a patient or family member. Prepare to tell the story.

**Take a gurney ride:** Wearing a patient gown, get taken on a gurney ride by a transporter from the emergency room to a distant inpatient room. Look, listen, feel.

**Conduct visitor interviews:** Walk visitors to their cars and find out what they experienced during their visit. Encourage them to share their observations, concerns, and anxieties.

**Take photographs:**
- Take a walk through the organization, looking through a patient's eyes.
- Identify ten visible indications that patients are not front and center.

- Take photographs of these ten visible indicators. These may be, for example, user-unfriendly signs, awkward room arrangements, confusing instructions, and messes.

**Share stories of the patients' experiences of caring:**
- On patient rounds, ask patients and families to describe in detail the absolute best experience they had in your organization.
- Ask for permission to share it with others.
- Collect all leaders' write-ups, edit them as needed, and produce a simple magazine for all leaders and staff.

**Create an anxiety map:** Have each leader make a map of one service process for which they are responsible. Have them identify at each step the patient's likely anxieties.

**Be a transporter-in-training:**
- Borrow a transporter uniform.
- Spend ninety minutes with a transporter as that transporter's trainee.
- Note the *patients'* experience. How do the patients see transport and nursing interacting? How long do the patients have to wait? What do the patients experience as they are taken to an ancillary service area? What are their likely anxieties?

**Zoom in on one step:** Experience one step in a service process the way several patients experience it.
- Identify a high-traffic point where patients come for service.
- Sit in that area in an inconspicuous place, reading a magazine.
- Listen and notice. What are patients experiencing at that point in a service? What anxieties and concerns are they likely to have? Where are the opportunities to improve that patient experience?

**Shadow a patient:** Experience one service fully.
- Ask a patient if you can tag along so you can try to see the experience through the patient's eyes.
- After shadowing, interview the patient on what helped reduce their anxiety and build their confidence.

**Eavesdrop:** In an area where staff make follow-up calls to patients, arrange for each leader to listen in on three of these calls (with permission from and full disclosure to staff and patients) in order to learn about patients' experiences and needs.

**Conduct a close-to-home interview:** Interview one of your own loved ones who was a patient in a service within the organization. Find out in detail the story of his or her experience.

The challenge with any of these exercises is to keep your focus on the experience of the patient, *not* on identifying and solving problems.

Maintaining a patient perspective in the face of so much to do and using self-discipline to adopt a posture of empathy take focus, commitment, and practice. It's not easy, but there's a payoff: when you do get things done, your actions will be grounded in your empathy for patients and your understanding of their experience.

• • •

# Additional Tools

## Tool 1
## PATIENT EXPERIENCE INTERVIEWS

Hand these questions out to your team.

- Ask each person to use the questions to interview three patients and/or family members over the course of the week.
- Explain that you will reconvene to share results and insights, and set a date.

When you reconvene, ask your team:

- What did you learn?
- What points caught your interest or curiosity?
- How might this inform how we proceed in our work? What themes do you see?
- Other sharing?

---

**Directions for Patient Experience Interviews**

1. Sit with the person. Get yourself present and adopt a curious attitude.
2. Explain (address the person by name), "You may know that we, the staff at_____ , are currently working on communicating our empathy more effectively and consistently with our patients and families. We want you to feel cared for, supported, and special. I'm hoping that you might be willing to answer a few questions to help us engage in this process with more understanding. Would it be okay if I ask you a few questions and take a few notes? Your name will remain confidential."
3. Say "Thank you!"
4. Take minimal notes during the interview, making sure you return frequently to sustain eye contact with the person.

1. Tell me about a time when you had a really positive experience with one of our staff. What happened, and specifically what made it such a positive experience for you?
2. What's really important for you to experience in your communication with staff here?
3. How well do you think I have (or another caregiver has) a sense of who you are (or your loved one who is a patient here) as a person? How can you tell?
4. If you could have a "dream" therapist (nurse, doctor, etc.), what would that person be like (name qualities)? How would he or she treat you (probe for specifics)? What might that person say when he or she greets you?

## Tool 2
## REMEMBERING THE PATIENT PERSPECTIVE WHEN MAKING BUSINESS DECISIONS

If only the patient were always in the room. We would be more self-conscious and patient conscious when we are making planning and financial decisions.

Here are two ways to help your team remember to consider the patient perspective:

- **BWATP.** Make a plaque or sign that says "BWATP." It stands for "But what about the patient!?" Post this in meeting rooms, and invite everyone to point to the sign when decisions need to be checked for their impact on patients.
- **Pat, the patient.** Have you seen the life-size stuffed people dolls? Have one made and dress it up in a patient gown. Have your team name this "patient." Plant your patient in a seat in meeting rooms, and invite people to point to Herb or Pat when they think the discussion needs to be informed by or checked for the patient perspective.

# Chapter 2

• • •

# Lessening Patient Anxiety

*Many patients experience anxiety. Help your staff to reduce or even eliminate it by improving systems and developing anxiety-reducing communications.*

For years, very little research was available about outpatient satisfaction. Because the services—physical therapy, radiology, visits with an internist—differed in substance, researchers believed there was little point in studying satisfaction with any one type of outpatient service. Also, because in outpatient services the relationship between caregiver and patient is typically short term, hospitals tended to see little promise in enhancing satisfaction and few opportunities to do so.

Now, with so many services delivered on an outpatient basis and so much revenue associated with these services, we've come to care very much about optimizing outpatient satisfaction. Fortunately, a plethora of commercially available surveys, as well as the Consumer Assessment of Healthcare Providers and Systems surveys, help us measure satisfaction in medical practices, health plans, and varied outpatient services.

Of all the research on outpatient services, the most powerful is many years old and comes from Philadelphia's Thomas Jefferson University Hospital. In the 1980s, Jefferson marketing experts saw the wave of the future in outpatient services and decided to investigate the factors affecting outpatient satisfaction. Using intensive interviews and focus groups, their study revealed a very important finding.

Regardless of the type of service, the attribute most highly correlated with outpatient satisfaction is "the extent to which staff made an effort to reduce my anxiety." When staff take steps to prevent or reduce patient anxiety, patients appreciate it. There's nothing shocking about this. Yet its practical implications have not been fully tapped.

## Reducing Anxiety

Lessons learned from research on outpatient satisfaction apply to the inpatient experience as well. For both outpatient and inpatient services, we can include deliberate ways to prevent or reduce patient anxiety throughout all service processes. We can find out from patients and families which steps of the service make them anxious. We can learn about the nature of their anxieties. Then we can engage our teams in dreaming up and installing design features (process steps, scripts, and communications) to prevent or reduce predictable anxiety.

Fortunately, it's easy to engage staff in anxiety-reduction strategies. Everyone understands anxiety, and health care professionals have enough empathy and personal experience to imagine the anxieties that their patients/customers are likely to feel at different steps of the service process.

In the chart below are foreseeable anxieties and some actions that can lessen or eliminate them.

| | |
|---|---|
| Patients wonder when they will get their test results. | Build into the process consistently delivered, clear information about when and how they will receive these results. |
| Patients anticipating certain tests worry about how much they will hurt. | Plan an effective way to adjust their expectations, alerting them accurately to the pain involved. |
| Patients asked to change into a robe worry about their valuables. | Make sure they know what to do with their valuables, or provide a system for protecting them. |
| Anxious family members will want information about their loved one in an intensive care unit. | Give a personal identification number to the people allowed to get patient updates so that nurses can safely give confidential information. |
| A parent leaving the pediatrician's office worries about what to do if the child's symptoms become worse. | Ensure that the caregiver consistently explains exactly how the parent can access help during off hours. |

*(Continued on next page)*

| | |
|---|---|
| Family members of a very sick loved one have trouble leaving after visiting hours. | Systematically tell them that caregivers will pay close attention and take good care, and give them a number they can call if they find themselves wakeful and anxious. |
| Patients become nervous at the end of shift, wondering if the next nurse will take good care of them. | Have a script for a nurse to express confidence in the night-shift colleague and reassure the patient that the next nurse will take great care. |

*Great* service is designed. One constructive approach to service design involves tuning in to the anxieties of patients and families, then consciously and conscientiously building into our everyday processes targeted methods and communications that head off or reduce anxiety.

## How Managers Can Engage Their Teams

Here's one way a manager can work with a team to make service improvements that will reduce customer anxiety.

1. Map the process for your service. What does the patient experience first, second, and third?
2. At each step, talk to patients and families. Learn the anxieties that arise with each step in the process.
3. Brainstorm ways to prevent anxiety that you now know to expect.
4. Brainstorm ways to reduce anxiety that you can't fully prevent.
5. Answer these fruitful questions:
   - What could a staff member say to relieve the patient's or family member's anxiety?
   - What improvement could prevent or relieve anxiety at that step in the process?
6. Focus on execution. Build the above steps into the process as a consistent, reliable part of the service.

## Team Exercise: Anxiety Reduction Worksheet

| Steps along the service process: | Likely anxieties during this step: | Your anxiety-reducing ideas:<br>• What can staff do or say to prevent anxiety?<br>• What can staff do or say to relieve anxiety? |
|---|---|---|
| | | |
| | | |
| | | |

## An Example from Volunteer Services Department

| Step along the service process | Likely anxieties during this step | How to reduce this anxiety |
|---|---|---|
| • Family sitting in surgery waiting room | • Anxiety about loved one's progress and condition<br>• Waiting as every minute feels like an hour | • Every thirty minutes a nurse liaison goes to surgical suite, talks to nurses and the surgeon, and reports back to family spokesperson with an update |

This next simple worksheet guides staff in using the anxiety-reduction approach to develop scripts for everyday situations.

## Service Mapping Worksheet

Step in customer's pathway through the service:

Likely anxieties at this step:

Suggested script that relieves or prevents anxiety:

Using the anxiety-reduction concept to drive service improvement is easy to explain and easy to do. That makes it refreshing. Introduce it to your management team at a staff meeting, and try it out then and there. Then encourage managers, grounded in that successful experience, to use it with their teams.

● ● ●

# Additional Tools

### Tool 1
### THE LINK PLAN: IMPROVING THE HANDOFF PROCESS WITH ANXIETY MAPPING

To identify improvements in handoffs, focus your team on what's happening at the end of one step in the service pathway and between that step and the next. Then design a link plan outlining anxiety-reducing words and behaviors that are key during the transition.

This plan should include:

● Informing the customer about what's happening and what can be expected
● Addressing customer anxieties with empathy and concern
● Showing them the way
● Making sure they have everything with them that they and the next service provider need
● Introducing or orienting the customer to the person or service on the receiving end
● Saying a gracious goodbye with a good wish and a smile

At every moment, the patient/customer should feel clear, secure, and confident that, with the person/service on the receiving end, he or she will be in good hands.

To organize a discussion with your staff, carve out a few important and connected steps in your customer's service pathway. In the chart below, write in the steps in the pathway.

Then, with your team, discuss and fill in the customer's likely anxieties at each step, *and during the transition from each step to the next,* the customer's likely questions and concerns.

|  | Step 1 | Step 2: Transition | Step 3 | Step 4: Transition | Step 5 |
|---|---|---|---|---|---|
| Likely customer anxieties |  |  |  |  |  |
| Likely customer questions |  |  |  |  |  |
| Important communication points |  |  |  |  |  |
| Important behavior and words for making handoff |  |  |  |  |  |
| What to take with them |  |  |  |  |  |

Then, focusing on one transition at a time, with the customer's likely anxieties and questions in mind, identify the key behaviors, message points, handouts, forms, and the like that should systematically occur or are needed during the transition between that step and the next.

## *Tool 2*
## LEADING THE PATIENT FROM PLACE TO PLACE: ONE EXAMPLE OF AN ANXIETY-REDUCING TRANSITION

This example applies to a mammography service. The goal: for the tech to lead the patient from the reception area to the changing cubicle in a way that reduces the woman's anxiety.

| Link Plan | Transition: Tech approaches patient in waiting area and escorts to changing area |
|---|---|
| What to take with them? | • Patient chart, information sheet, etc. |
| Likely patient anxieties | • Will this person be nice?<br>• Will the gown cover me?<br>• Will this be private?<br>• Will my belongings be safe?<br>• How badly will this hurt?<br>• Do I have breast cancer? |
| Likely patient questions | • How much do I have to disrobe?<br>• How long will I have to wait for the tech to arrive?<br>• How long will it take me to get the results? |
| Important communication points that anticipate and address these anxieties and questions (main points and/or exact words) | • Greet warmly and call person by preferred name. "Hello, Mrs. Harold. I'm glad to see you again."<br>• "Let me show you the way to the changing area."<br>• "Now, let me explain a bit for you."<br>• "This outer room is *private*. No one will come in until you hear me knock to see if you're ready."<br>• "I'm giving you this nice roomy robe and will give you privacy to put it on in the cubicle."<br>• "You'll need to remove everything above the waist. It's fine to keep your slacks and shoes on."<br>• "When you're ready, come out and have a seat right here. You can leave your belongings in the cubicle. They'll be safe there. But of course, if you prefer to bring your purse, that's fine."<br>• "I'll knock after a few minutes to see if you're ready, and then we'll move into this other room for your mammogram."<br>• "Now, before I go, what questions or concerns do you have? I want you to feel informed and comfortable." |

Your team can create the link plan together by committee or in a staff meeting. Best approach: have two different pairs of people work on each transition point, and then compare notes and make improvements that build on the strengths in each pair's link plan.

# Chapter 3

• • •

# A Giant Step toward
# Patient-Centered Care

*Care-full explanations make good intentions explicit,
provide realistic expectations, and relieve anxiety.*

Reaching the next level of superior service is less about making patients happy and more about communicating our compassion and easing patient anxiety. That's what makes our mission distinct from that of Disney or the Ritz-Carlton.

To create breakthroughs in communicating compassion and easing anxiety, we need to do some hard work on the nature and quality of the explanations our care teams give to patients and their families.

Patient satisfaction surveys typically include questions like the ones below, and the answers provide insight into how well our teams are performing one pivotally important task—explaining:

- "Did the nurse or physician explain?"
- "Did they explain in a way you could understand?"
- "Did they tell you what you could expect?"
- "Did you receive discharge instructions?"
- "Did they invite your questions?"
- "Were options explained to you?"

Most hospital patients feel out of their element, perhaps frightened, anxious, impatient, or overwhelmed. To give them a sense of control, relieve their anxiety, and reduce the mystery associated with complex hospital care, they rely on their caregivers to explain.

And, while better-quality explanations from health care staff have a well-documented effect on patient satisfaction, they also result in more positive health outcomes. When an explanation reduces the patients' anxiety, increases their sense of control, and builds confidence in their caregivers, patients are more likely to absorb information, cooperate in their care, follow the caregivers' advice, and feel less anxious. This frees up energy for treatment and healing.

## Strategies for Giving Care-Full Explanations

Many organizations have worked on standardizing explanations of clinical facts; plans and choices; discharge instructions; and other clinical, technical, and task-related information. But truly great explanations address more than the tasks and actions at hand. They address the affective domain—feelings, anxieties, and concerns. And few caregiver teams have invested the necessary time and attention to designing the affective elements of great explanations and standardizing their use in patient care. It is these elements that make the caregiver's caring nature glaringly clear to patients and families.

### The Six Consequences of Care-Less Explanations

- Mystery
- Misunderstandings
- Misgivings
- Mistrust
- Misfortune
- Missed opportunities

Targeting the quality of explanations as a service improvement priority can create breakthroughs in the patient experience. Here are six strategies for providing more *care-full* explanations to patients and their families.

### Avoiding Mystery: Care-Full Explanations Address Feelings, Anxieties, and Concerns—The Heart, Not Just the Head

While thoroughly explaining what you're doing in words people can understand is important and basic, care-full explanations address far more than the tasks, activities, and procedures that consume people's task-oriented minds.

## Patient-Centered Explanations

- Make the caregiver's good intentions explicit.
- Adjust expectations so they are realistic.
- Address the spoken and unspoken anxieties of patients and families.

### Avoiding Misunderstandings: Patient-Centered Explanations Make the Caregiver's Good Intentions Clear

We know that our team members have good, caring intentions. They mean well as they care for patients. But the patient doesn't necessarily perceive their caring intentions, because caregivers frequently explain their action as an end in itself. "I'm here to take your vital signs now," instead of "I want to check on how you're doing, make sure all is OK. I'm here to take your vital signs." Here are more examples.

## Explanations with and without Positive Intent

| Without Expressed Positive Intent | Unintended Negative Impact | With Positive Intent Expressed |
|---|---|---|
| "Let's review these instructions." | The patient can think, "Does she think I'm stupid?" | "Do you mind if I review these instructions? I want to be sure I've been clear so you will feel confident that you know what to do." |
| "Please push the call button sooner next time." | The patient might feel judged or chastised. | "I want to be here for you when you need me. It would be a big help to me if you could call for me earlier." |
| "Please hold the line for a moment." | The caller feels neglected or unimportant. | "I want to be sure I'm giving you the right number. Would you mind holding for a moment?" |
| "Visiting hours are over. You'll need to leave." | The family is annoyed and feels the policy serves the hospital, not them. | "It's getting late and I want some privacy with your dad to help him prepare for a restful night. So how about going home and getting some rest yourself? You've been so supportive, and it can be exhausting." |

A care-full explanation makes the caregiver's positive intent explicit and reflects what's good *for the patient*.

### Avoiding Misgivings: Patient-Centered Explanations Ensure Expectations Are Realistic

Unrealistic expectations on the part of patients and their families are the seeds that grow into anxiety, complaints, and dissatisfaction. "How dare they keep me waiting so long? Why are they taking people before me who came in after me? Did they forget about telling me my test results?" If we tell people up front how long things are going to take, how much pain they are likely to experience and how we can help them with it, when they can expect results, and why, we make it possible for them to adapt, knowing that their care is progressing as expected and that we want them to feel informed and secure.

| Patient's Expectation before Adjustment | Explanation to Adjust the Expectation |
|---|---|
| Patient in emergency department expects to be taken in order of arrival. | "I want you to know up front that we have three teams providing different types of care. You might see others who arrived after you called in before you are. That could mean one of two things: Either they are being helped by a team different from the one you need, or their health issue is higher risk and needs more urgent attention. Thanks for understanding." |
| Patient arrives for appointment and expects to be taken immediately. | "I want to alert you to the fact that the doctor is running late, and your wait is likely to be about forty-five minutes. Some patients required more time than we estimated. And the doctor gives all patients the time they need." |

### Avoiding Mistrust: Patient-Centered Explanations Address Patient and Family Anxiety

When caregivers stop to think about it, they can easily identify likely anxieties of patients. After all, caregivers have seen many patients going through similar procedures, illnesses, courses of treatment, emotional swings, and the like. Even when a patient does not express anxiety, observant caregivers can address it with sensitivity. For example:

| Patient's Likely Anxiety | Explanation to Ease Anxiety |
|---|---|
| Worry about postsurgery pain | "You might be wondering about the pain after your surgery. I want to ease your mind about this. Here's our plan." |
| Worry about being forgotten when nurse leaves at change of shift | "I'll be leaving in a half hour. Nancy Smith is taking over for me, and she is terrific. And I will be sure to pass along to her the important events of your day. You'll be in very good hands with Nancy." |

## Avoiding Misfortune: You Said It, But Did They Get It?

Care-full explanations are explanations that are understood by the recipient. No matter how well crafted, an explanation fails unless the person hearing it comprehends it.

It isn't adequate to ask, "Do you understand?" The patient's answer tells you nothing because people may be afraid to admit that they don't understand, or they might not realize they don't understand. You have no clue about what they have understood.

| To Check Understanding, Say | Don't Say |
|---|---|
| "I've said a lot, and I'm concerned that I might not have been clear. What is your understanding of the most important things to do once you get home?" | "Do you understand?" |
| "This information can feel overwhelming. What questions do you have at this point? I really want to address them." | "Are you clear?" |

 An explanation is incomplete until the communicator respectfully checks understanding.

## Avoiding Missed Opportunities: Care-Full Explanations Are Designed and Delivered Consistently

To many frontline caregivers, scripts that dictate the exact words they must say are abhorrent. If they don't want to follow a script verbatim, they can identify essential message points or "key elements" that they can deliver in their own words. The point is that caregivers cannot produce consistently great explanations unless they design the key message points and cover these message points consistently. These elements need to address not only the facts but also the patient's anxieties, feelings, and concerns.

Here's a worksheet that work teams can use to develop care-full explanations for their everyday situations.

## Key Words Worksheet

| Communication Need | Great Key Words |
|---|---|
| Acknowledge likely anxiety. | |
| Express positive intent. | |
| Adjust expectations. | |

For example, notice below that all three functions are served sequentially in one well-designed explanation.

## Explanation of the Discharge Process

| Communication Need | Great Key Words |
|---|---|
| Acknowledge likely anxiety. | "I realize you might be impatient to go home, and now that the doctor said you can go, you want to get on your way." |
| Express positive intent. | "When you leave, I want you to feel well prepared and safe, and I want to help you on your way as quickly as possible. I want you to know what the discharge process entails. There's quite a lot to it." |
| Adjust expectations. | "The discharge process takes up to __ hours because there are so many things that need to be done. Here's what they are and why they need to be done before you go . . . I really appreciate your understanding." |

# Taking Caring Communication to the Next Level

Albert Einstein said, "Excellence is in the details." Service excellence is achievable only if we lead our teams through the hard work of designing explanations that address not only the cognitive but also the affective domain. Until we do that, patients will remain fearful, and care will not feel supportive and personal. Our patients deserve better.

• • •

# Additional Tools

## Tool 1
### CARE-FULL EXPLANATIONS: FIVE EXAMPLES FOR THE EMERGENCY DEPARTMENT

| | |
|---|---|
| 1. Waiting room rounds | • "Hello, Mr. Vasquez, my name is Sam Simms, and I'm a patient representative (volunteer, nurse) here in the emergency room."<br>• "I'm here to check on you and to let you know that we haven't forgotten about you."<br>• "I'm so sorry about the wait. I can assure you we haven't forgotten about you."<br>• "As far as your wait, I've checked with the nurse, and she estimates that it will be about ___ minutes/hours."<br>• "How are you doing? Is there anything I can do to make you more comfortable?"<br>• "Thank you for your patience." |
| 2. If patient or companion asks why or complains that others have been taken first | • "We want to give everyone the care they need, and different patients need different kinds of care. Some patients are better cared for in our Fast Track area. Others need our acute care area. So sometimes, someone who came after you needs a different kind of care and gets taken first. Also, we have a practice of taking the people who are in greatest danger first. I really appreciate your understanding." |
| 3. If patient has concern about stepping away to bathroom or phone | • "I want to assure you that we won't forget about you. If for some reason you don't hear the nurse call your name, maybe because you're in the bathroom or dozing, the nurse will move on to the next person and then call your name again next." |
| 4. Triage nurse—periodic check on patient while in reception area | • "Mr. Vasquez, I want to check on how you're doing."<br>• Make eye contact, smile. Move to patient's level. Make caring, concerned expression.<br>• "How are you feeling?"<br>• "Let me do a quick check of a few things . . . (your temperature, etc.)"<br>• "I'm sorry about the wait. It looks like it will be about ___ more minutes."<br>• "Is there anything I can do to make you more comfortable while you wait?"<br>• "Thank you for your patience." |

*(Continued on next page)*

| 5. Waiting for an inpatient room | • **Be proactive. Tell them what they can expect and why:** "The process here has many steps in it. For that reason, it usually takes about (time estimate) before we can locate the right type of room for you and prepare that room by cleaning it and getting the right supplies delivered."<br>• **Apologize and empathize:** "(Name), I'm sorry you're still waiting. I realize it's so frustrating to wait when you came here to see a doctor."<br>• **State your positive intent:** "I assure you I will do all I can to take you in quickly."<br>• **Explain:** "The problem is, for reasons I hope you'll understand, our policy is to take people in life-threatening situations ahead of people with problems that can wait. Also, because this is a teaching hospital, we have our physicians and residents talk with you and examine you, which also take time. What's more, there may be waits because of the tests the doctor will think you need. Then, after all of that is done, we need to find an appropriate room for you and go through the process of preparing it for you. This too can take awhile, since the patient in the room before you might take more time than we expected to vacate the room."<br>• **Revise time estimate:** "So getting you to a room might take as long as _____."<br>• **Offer options:** In the meantime, can I get you something to make you more comfortable? Would you like to use a phone, read a magazine . . . ?"<br>• **Say thanks again and that you appreciate the patient:** "OK, thanks for staying and waiting. We really appreciate your patience." |
|---|---|

*Tool 2*
# A PATIENT-FRIENDLY FACT SHEET TO ADDRESS ANXIETY AND ADJUST EXPECTATIONS

This fact sheet explains how the emergency department (ED) works. But more than that, it addresses anxieties likely in patients and their companions who unhappily find themselves in the ED. It also helps to adjust expectations, so patients and their companions will be a tad more understanding about what is so often a very frustrating process for them.

---

## Welcome to the Emergency Room!

Because being in the Emergency Room is something you didn't plan for and also might be a new experience for you, the Emergency Room team wants you to know about how the Emergency Room works and what you can expect.

Our Emergency Room (ER) is open 24 hours a day, 7 days a week, and 365 days a year. Our skilled doctors, nurses, and assistants are on hand to handle a wide range of medical problems. We will do our best to make sure that you are taken care of with respect, sensitivity, and dignity.

### What Can You Expect?

1. First, when you arrive, we will ask you to register at one of our patient registration windows. Our registration clerk will ask you your name and address and why you are here.
   - If you have an immediate and urgent medical emergency, your clerk will call the charge nurse to arrange for you to be seen immediately by our care team. Or,
   - If you can safely wait, your clerk will ask you to have a seat in the reception area until the triage nurse comes for you. The triage nurse will come for you in a few minutes (usually within a half-hour).
2. The next person you will meet is the triage nurse. The triage nurse will ask you questions about why you're here, your medical history, medications, and allergies. This nurse might also record your vital signs such as temperature, pulse, and blood pressure. Based on what the triage nurse learns, he or she will arrange for you to see the right person on our team.

---

3.  After talking with the triage nurse, patients need to complete registration. We do bedside registration later for patients who have a life-threatening condition. For others, we ask you to return to the registration window and speak again with a clerk. The clerk will ask you a few more questions, including your insurance information. This is necessary so we can develop a medical record where we will keep all information we collect about your condition. *Please know that we will treat you whether or not you have insurance.*

4.  Based on your illness or injury, the registration clerk will either ask you to have a seat again in the reception area or arrange for you to be taken directly into the treatment area.

5.  When it's time for you to go to one of our treatment areas, the charge nurse will come for you in the reception area and take you there.

***How Long Will You Have to Wait?*** We realize it's hard to wait when you don't feel well or are in pain. While we will do our best to make sure that you are taken care of as quickly as possible, many people unfortunately have to wait quite a long time, sometimes several hours. Why might there be a long wait?

- **We are sometimes overcrowded.** An emergency room does not schedule appointments. We have no control over how many patients arrive at a given time. You may arrive at an especially busy time and have to wait because of that.

- **We don't follow a "take a number" system.** Sometimes, you will think, "I'm next," but still have to wait.

    —**Our team sees patients in an order determined by how severe their problem is.** We care first for people with the most critical medical needs. For example, a patient having a heart attack might be seen before another patient with a less life-threatening need. If your situation is less urgent, you may have to wait longer. That's why people with less urgent needs often choose to go to a doctor's office instead of an emergency room.

    —**We take care of many patients who come by ambulance.** They are wheeled in through a door that goes directly to the treatment area—a door you can't see from the reception area. These people are in life-or-death situations and demand immediate attention.

—**We are channeling people to four different treatment areas.**
We have four different treatment areas: Trauma (for severe
emergencies), Urgent (for people with less severe emergencies),
Observation (for people who need to be watched very closely), and
Fast Track (for people who have health issues that are not urgent
or complicated). Sometimes, we take someone else before you
because they are going to a different treatment area than you.

While you're waiting, take a few minutes to jot down everything you
want to tell the doctor. Also, list your questions. This will make it
easier for you when you see the doctor.

**Who Will Take Care of You?** Our Emergency Room takes a team
approach to patient care. Nurses, techs, medical students, resident
physicians, and attending physicians all have a part in evaluation,
treatment, and care. Every patient has an attending physician who
creates their care plan and coordinates their care.

### What Happens in the Treatment Area?

- A nurse will start your treatment process, asking you questions and
  perhaps asking you to change into a hospital gown.
- The nurse will lead you to a place inside the treatment area where
  you can relax as much as possible until the doctor comes to see you.
  Hopefully, there will be a room available for you. Sometimes, when all
  the rooms are full, we provide a bed in the hallway. And sometimes,
  if all of the hallway beds are full, we provide a chair for you where we
  can check in on you and make sure you're safe until the doctor can
  see you. We know it's very frustrating and inconvenient for patients
  and their loved ones when no rooms or beds are available. But our
  space is limited, and we really appreciate your understanding as we
  do our best to care for you.
- The nurse might also connect you to a device (a monitor) that
  makes it possible for us to watch your vital signs.
- In a half-hour or so, one of our ER doctors will come to talk with you.
  He or she will take a more complete medical history and examine
  you. The doctor then diagnoses your problem or orders tests to help
  in the diagnosis. Please tell the doctor how you feel, exactly what's
  bothering you, and if you are in pain. Don't hesitate to speak up, and
  don't hesitate to ask questions.

***What If You Need Tests or X-Rays?*** The doctor will order any lab tests or x-rays that you might need. The ER has its own x-ray room, but you may be taken to another department for other special studies. We might send a sample of your blood and urine to the lab for testing. While you are waiting for your test results, please let the nurse know if you are in pain or if your symptoms change. Tell a nurse if you need any help. Also, please do not eat or drink anything until you check with your nurse.

***Can Your Family Stay with You?*** This all depends on how crowded we are, whether there is space, and whether you want or need privacy. Usually, both parents may stay with a sick or injured child. And usually, an adult patient may have one or two family members or friends stay with them in the treatment area. There may be times when we ask family or friends to leave the treatment area so that our care team can best do our job.

***Will There Be More Waiting in the Treatment Area?*** Probably yes. If you need observation, that takes time. If you need tests or treatments, we have to arrange for skilled staff and equipment, and we might have to request a transporter to take you to the right place for the test or treatment. Once your tests and treatments are done, technologists have to analyze the results and communicate them to your doctor. If you are having several tests, the doctor needs to wait for all of the results, so he or she has the whole picture of what is going on. Then the doctor studies the results and comes to talk to you. There are many steps and many people involved in your care. While we're very busy behind the scenes, you are waiting and waiting, and that's very hard. Let our nursing team know if they can do anything to make you more comfortable during this time. They'll be glad to.

***Then What Happens?*** After you have received a diagnosis and, if needed, emergency care, the doctor will make a decision about your discharge. One of three things will happen: You will be admitted to the hospital. Or you will be discharged to go home. Or you will be referred to another facility suited to your needs. The doctor will discuss this decision.

- **What if you have to stay in the hospital?** If you do need to be admitted to the hospital, because our hospital is so often full, you might have to wait for a hospital room to become open. As soon as your room is ready, the ER nurse will give your report and treatment plan to the nurse on your new hospital unit. One of our escorts will take you to your hospital room, where you will be greeted by a nurse.

- **What if the doctor says you can go home?** If the doctor discharges you, members of our care team will make sure you have follow-up instructions. Don't be shy about asking questions. Make sure you know exactly what you need to do after you leave, symptoms to watch for, medications to take, and more. We want you to feel confident and clear about next steps for you. If you need follow-up care and you don't have your own doctor, we will refer you to one.

## We Want Your Feedback!

Several days after your emergency room visit, you might be one of the people randomly selected to receive a confidential survey that asks you to evaluate your experience in our emergency room. If you receive a Patient Satisfaction Survey, please, please, please fill it out and return it, so we can learn about your experience and also make improvements.

*As you can see, a visit to an emergency room*
*is an experience! We want to make your visit with us*
*positive and healing. Thank you for coming to us.*
*Thank you for your understanding.*
*We wish you well.*

# Chapter 4

• • •

# Using Scripts for
# Patient Interactions

*Staff members often oppose standardized
statements for communicating with patients,
but authentic use of well-designed words
can greatly improve patient satisfaction.*

Call the Ritz-Carlton right now. Ask any question. After you hear
the answer, say, "Thank you." You'll hear the Ritz person say warmly,
"My pleasure!"

"My pleasure." It's a script. It's a script that the Ritz folks learn
during new employee orientation, practice during their first day on
the job, and use consistently from then on.

Left to their own devices, Ritz employees, like employees every-
where, would utter various and sundry words in their own particular
styles. Some might say, "You're welcome," or "No problem," or "Hold,
please," or "Don't mind a bit." But at the Ritz-Carlton, their super-
visors tell them that the words to respond to a customer's "thanks"
are "my pleasure." And the Ritz gets extremely high customer satisfaction for this and many other well-scripted interactions.

Consider health care. Many employees are ambivalent about or
downright resistant to scripts. They offer plenty of reasons not to
use them, and while there is a grain of truth in their retorts, none of
these is a good enough reason to resist:

- "Scripts sound mechanical." Scripts don't have to sound mechanical. With practice and clear expectations, staff can learn to sound
  authentic.

- "My staff hate scripts, and I can't afford to make them angry because I need every warm body I can get." Staff members may not like the idea of scripts initially, but they'll be happier if you help them deal effectively with patients.
- "Scripts make everyone sound alike." With scripts, there is room for diverse styles. Different people should be allowed to tailor the scripts to their style if it befits a professional and addresses all the message points that make a positive impression.
- "Who has time to work out scripts?" Who has time for anything nowadays? People make the time for what's important. And once staff are impressing customers, the customers are happier, more cooperative, and appreciative, and staff save time and prevent irritation.
- "Our people aren't good at the language they need to write good scripts." If you don't want to do scripting because you don't have people with the language skills to develop the scripts, then how in the world are they going to exhibit impressive behavior *without* scripts?

## You Don't Have a Choice

If you want your team to *impress* patients and other customers, then you have to implement scripts.

Consider stage actors and actresses. They start with a script, hopefully a good one, as well as stage directions that suggest behavior and feelings nonverbally. They read and reread the script to absorb its essence and make the words familiar. Then they think about how they will play it. They go to rehearsal, where their director sees their interpretation, gives feedback, and urges them to experiment with various approaches. Then they settle on a way to play it that seems most effective and impressive, rehearsing many times until the script is second nature. Finally, they walk on stage day after day to give a consistently credible performance, no matter how they feel. They might have problems at home, a headache, or a financial crisis, but they find a way to perform impeccably and please the audience night after night. Their performance is consistent, not mood dependent.

We can learn a lesson from them. In health care, too often, we create scripts; plop them on staff; and expect staff to use the scripts effectively, consistently, and immediately. We provide no experimenting with style, no rehearsals, and no coaching. After saying, "Just do it," is it any wonder that we breed resistance?

Staff who aren't naturals at great customer service need scripts, coaching, and rehearsals. It is managers who need to make this happen. They need to provide training, practice, and ongoing coaching if they want employees to make great scripts a habit, and they need to expect employees to perform with authenticity.

## The Manager's Role

The customers of every service follow a pathway through that service. There are key steps (*touch points*) along that pathway where employee behavior is critical. Managers need to create, acquire, or develop with employees words and body language that work at key touch points. Figure out the script that will ensure a memorable, positive customer experience at these and other touch points:

- During the first contact
- During a patient handoff from one staff member to another
- During a send-off or goodbye
- When telling customers what they can expect
- When adjusting customer expectations downward so they are realistic
- When explaining delays
- When checking for understanding
- When encouraging questions
- When dealing with a furious family member
- When dealing with an emotion-laden situation
- When wanting family members to feel included
- When communicating important messages that the patient doesn't want to hear
- When faced with a disrespectful doctor or colleague

## Service Mapping

Service mapping is a great tool that managers can use with staff to help them identify the touch points with patients or customers—touch points that they can make impressive through deliberate design and scripting. Here's the essence of service mapping:

- Draw a customer's pathway through a particular service.
- Interview customers at each step and ask them what makes them anxious or concerned at that particular step. You will hear

patterns: *many* people will feel the same concerns. For instance, when people are going to a changing room to disrobe before a test, they tend to experience specific anxieties ("What should I remove exactly? Will this robe cover me? Do I put it on front-ward or backward? Will my belongings be safe if I leave them here, or do I take them with me? Will others see me in this robe as I pass through the hallway? What will this test reveal?").

- Now that you know what causes anxiety for one customer after another, work with staff on *scripts* they can use at each step to anticipate customer feelings and concerns and *prevent* or *relieve* their anxiety. The script should anticipate each likely patient concern and address it before the patient has to ask or feel anxious about it.

| Anxiety Point | Staff Script |
|---|---|
| Patient might find waiting for results agonizing. | "I want you to know how long it takes to process this test and when you can expect the results. I realize that when you're waiting for results, minutes can feel like hours." |
| Patient might find so much information overwhelming. | "This is a lot for anyone to hear all at once. I'll go over it well and welcome your questions." |
| Patient fears appearing stupid. | "This is complicated, and I'm not always clear. What are the main points you heard in what I explained? I want to make sure I've been clear." |
| Patient fears forgetting what he or she is supposed to do. | "I can imagine that there may be a lot on your mind. Please don't hesitate to ask me to review anything you want to hear again." |

Are your patient satisfaction scores hitting the wall? Scripts that are well designed, thoroughly practiced, and well delivered, especially for high-anxiety interactions, can help you achieve breakthroughs. And there is no way to ensure consistently impressive customer service without scripts.

• • •

# Additional Tools

## Tool 1
## PRACTICE MAKES PERFECT
## WITH SCRIPT REHEARSAL

Service excellence requires rehearsal. Just as Broadway performers need to rehearse and refine their performances with the help of a coach or director, so, too, do hospital staff need to rehearse, perfect, and standardize *wow* approaches to their everyday customer interactions.

Challenge managers to engage their teams in rehearsing best practices so that they make them part of their everyday routines. It should be a default position that kicks in even in an atmosphere of bad moods, stress, and pressure.

### Rehearse Scripts

Engage high performers as performance coaches. Pair them up with individuals who need particular help.

- The manager meets with each individual in need of a coach and clarifies performance expectations (e.g., key words at key times are required to improve patient interactions).
- The manager offers to provide a performance coach—a peer who will help each individual polish his or her performance in a confidential way.

Round robin is a *very* quick process for helping people practice and perfect their behavior in everyday situations—like greetings, handoffs, apologizing for and explaining delays, and saying goodbye. Team members help each other perform better and better. The manager can run the round robin or engage a workshop facilitator or high performer to do so.

- Explain the purpose: to practice and become great in a particular situation with customers, so people can routinely perform in a great way.
- Have people line up double file, with partners facing each other, like so:

A    A    A    A    A

B    B    B    B    B

- People in row A try out their approach to the situation first, with the person in row B acting as the patient/customer.

  —Their partner/customer gives feedback and suggestions.

  —Then row A rotates, moving one step to the right, so that each person is opposite a new partner/customer. (The person at the far right end who doesn't now have a partner walks back to the other end of the line to find a new partner.)

  —The As try their best-practice approach with the new person B, this time using the feedback they received to perform even better. Their new partners give them feedback again.

  —Then the As rotate again. For the third time, they perform their best-practice approach, this time giving a really polished performance.

- Then, switch roles. The Bs are the performers and try their approach with their A partner/customer, following the same routine as above.

- At the end, convene the group and invite people to talk about what was hard, what was easy, and what advice they gave to others to maximize performance effectiveness.

- Mobilize staff to implement their polished approaches consistently. Make it clear that this is now a job expectation.

- Set a date for a check-up meeting.

## Tool 2
# ADVANCING SERVICE EXCELLENCE IN A MULTILINGUAL ENVIRONMENT

No doubt, your organization has employees or patients who don't speak English. And, no doubt, you are committed to these principles:

- No one should feel like a second-class citizen.
- No employee should be exempt from communicating in ways people can understand.

If this requires staff development, so be it. Take the high road by finding ways to communicate with every employee and patient, regardless of language.

When there are non-English-speaking people in significant numbers, what do you do?

- Go on record frequently about your commitment to cross-cultural communication and the importance of finding some way to understand and be understood across languages.

- Translate patient rights and responsibilities and the organization's mission and values into each of the languages spoken by large numbers of staff and patients. Frame these and hang them in a row (gallery-like) in a long hallway frequented by staff and visitors.
- Hire staff who are reflective of your patient populations so you have staff members who are fluent in the array of languages spoken by your patients.
- Provide on-site courses for employees in the languages most often spoken in the communities you serve.
- Mobilize interpretive services, using a mix of staff, volunteers, and fee-for-service interpreter services.
- Do more: institute simple scripts that allow some modicum of communication across language lines.

## Don't Hesitate to Script

Mobilize managers and their teams to work out basic scripts that connect patients and staff despite language barriers. Specifically, if you want to wow your patients:

- Expect employees to connect to patients and families in the patient's language.
- Expect employees who speak little English to connect in English with English-speaking patients.

Assume for the moment that you have patients and employees who speak only Spanish. Assume further that you have patients who speak only Spanish and staff who speak only English.

| A basic script for use by English-only workers with Spanish co-workers, patients, and families | (in Spanish)<br>• "Hello. My name is ____. I'm sorry I don't speak your language."<br>• "If you need help, I can find someone for you who will understand." |
|---|---|
| A basic script for use by Spanish-only workers with English-only co-workers, patients, and families | (in English)<br>• "Good morning. Nice to see you. (Smiling) I'm sorry I don't speak English."<br>• "If you need anything, I will be happy to find your nurse for you."<br>• "What else can I do for you?"<br>• "Are you satisfied with my service today?"<br>• "Good day to you." |

## Diversify Your Staff Development Methods

While we want to primarily employ people who speak some English, sometimes this is impossible. To send a message that service excellence is for everyone and to give a respectful message of inclusion, take extra steps to involve non-English-speaking people in your service strategy.

| | |
|---|---|
| Materials | Print in English on the right-hand page and in the other language on the left-hand page facing it. |
| Sessions | Hold some sessions in the other language and/or engage some bilingual facilitators. |
| Promotional materials and campaigns | When you produce awareness-raising materials, such as posters, include both languages. |
| Multiple languages | If there are several languages dominant in your organization, pick the three that relate to the most people and do the above for all three. |

These extra measures go a long way toward creating a culture of inclusion that sends a powerful message of respect to your diverse team and the people and communities you serve.

# Chapter 5

• • •

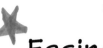

# Easing the Wait
# for Patients

*Staff can lessen anxiety and resentment
by keeping patients informed, explaining the reason
for the delay, and providing diversions.*

You know from experience that when a person is worried, sick, pressured, nervous, in pain, bored, uncomfortable, hungry, restless, or fearful, every minute of waiting feels like an hour. Waiting for appointments, waiting to see the doctor, waiting for results, waiting for a callback, waiting for an answer, waiting, waiting, waiting—all kinds of waits are irritating and stir resentment toward the care team. Just eavesdrop in a waiting room for a few minutes, and you'll hear, "They think their time is more valuable than mine! They have no respect for my time!"

Advances in technology have destroyed what little tolerance people had for waiting under these circumstances. E-mail, voice mail, fax, Federal Express, Priority Mail, instant messaging, high-speed Internet, and the like have changed people's expectations. We want it now.

Growing impatience makes it awfully difficult to achieve and sustain patient satisfaction. As consumers become understandably and increasingly demanding, speed has become a powerful competitive factor in patient satisfaction.

What are we to do?

## The Psychology of Waiting

When people are waiting, they are under a lot of stress. *The Service Encounter,* edited by J. Czepiel (Lexington Books, 1984), talks about an entire psychology of waiting. Consider these facts about waiting, along with ideas to reduce the stress:

*Anxiety makes waiting seem longer.* We need to figure out words and ways to reduce anxiety. For example:

- "If you need to use the restroom, don't hesitate. You won't lose your turn."
- "If you need to let someone know how long you'll be, you're welcome to use this phone or your cell phone."
- "Would you like to read a magazine?"

*Waits of uncertain length are harder to tolerate.* Too often, staff members say nothing about the upcoming wait because they are embarrassed about it or they don't know how to estimate it. Nevertheless, we need to write scripts that staff can use to advise patients of the waiting time. For instance, "The doctor will be able to see you within twenty minutes." Or "It can take up to four hours before the doctor can see you because some procedures take unexpectedly long periods of time."

*Waiting feels longer when you don't know the reason for the wait.* People sit there stewing when we don't explain why we're keeping them waiting. We need to make regular updates by staff a routine, not an afterthought. "Mrs. Jones, I realize you've been waiting for nearly two hours. I'm really sorry. I want to explain and give you an update. We've had ambulances bring in trauma victims through another entrance. These people have needed a lot of our staff's attention because they are in life-or-death situations. I'm sorry this has meant that you're waiting a long time. At this point, I'm estimating that it could be another ninety minutes."

*People are much less tolerant when their wait feels unfair.* Let patients know why they're waiting longer than others: "Mr. Hardy, I want to explain why some people who arrived after you might be taken before you. People in this area are here for three different services. You will be taken when the team that provides the specific service you came for is ready. In the meantime, some other services might be ready for the other people, who are here for those services. So they are taken before you."

*The more valuable the service, the longer a person is willing to wait.* This is no excuse for being callous about keeping people waiting. Just because they lack alternative providers or want *this* doctor or *this* service doesn't make it acceptable to perpetuate long waits. Fix the flow to reduce the delays out of respect for the patients, even if the delays aren't causing you to lose business.

*Pre-process waits feel much longer than in-process waits.* It's important to get the care process going, even if there will be delays along the way. Many emergency departments do bedside registration, have staging areas, or have triage nurses initiate tests immediately so that the person can be in process right away, even though there might then be long delays. In outpatient areas, people have an easier time waiting in the exam room than they do in the reception area because they feel that at least they are *in process.*

*Waiting alone feels longer than waiting in a group.* It helps the time pass if family and friends can keep a patient company during any delays. If you have a policy that prevents family and friends from joining patients in the exam room, reconsider it. Figure out a way to make it possible for other people to be with the patient.

*Occupied time feels shorter than unoccupied time.* When people don't have anything to do, the wait time feels longer. We need to use our considerable creativity and find ways to keep people occupied while they're waiting.

*If people think you feel really bad about inconveniencing them, they will be less angry at you.* We need to help the individuals on our teams eat humble pie and sincerely apologize to patients and families when we keep them waiting, no matter whose fault it is.

## Plan of Action

Here's my personal five-point plan for increasing respect for our customers' time.

 ## The Waiting List

1. Speed up the process.
2. Remove the term *waiting room* from all signs, literature, and people's vocabulary.
3. Provide diversions. Make the patient's time *feel* like it's going faster.
4. Adjust the customer's expectations. Underpromise and overdeliver.
5. Institute scripts and script rehearsal so that staff members use magic—not tragic—words when communicating with patients about delays.

Copyright ©2005 Wendy Leebov

*Speed up the process.* Eliminate or reduce delays through process and technology improvements. Use quality improvement processes to eliminate redundancies; limit the number of different people a patient has to interact with; reduce the distances patients have to travel; and locate all supplies, equipment, and forms at the caregivers' fingertips. Eliminate obsolete steps: hold a staff contest to find elements of the process that no longer serve a function. Acquire tools that work faster—faster computers, faster processing devices. Do flow analyses, and staff up at the logjam points. At its National Congress on Reducing Cycle Times and Delays, the Institute for Healthcare Improvement, Boston, shared terrific approaches. Bite the bullet and improve the process. It is not hopeless.

*Remove the term* waiting room *from all signs, literature, and people's vocabulary.* It sets up a negative expectation right from the start. How about calling it the Reception, Welcome, or Hospitality Area or some other creative, positive phrase that your employees suggest?

*Provide diversions. Make the patient's time* feel *like it's going faster.* Yesterday, as I sat waiting for an appointment, I asked fellow patients to brainstorm diversions with me. They suggested seek-and-find word games, brochures about the provider, a meet-the-staff bulletin board, Internet access, computer games, fish tanks, and more. My personal favorite for an emergency department (ED) reception area is an electronic bulletin board like those in bars—with news or trivia or programmed with messages about how the ED works, the strengths of the organization, child safety, wellness tips, and more. Inexpensive subscription services can make this very easy.

*Adjust the customer's expectations. Underpromise and overdeliver.* Discourage staff from predicting a wait length that is unrealistically short. Encourage staff to proactively shape the customer's expectations. Consider this: You call a bank for information and the banker says, "It will take some time to find the answer. I'll be back to you within twenty-four hours." Expecting it to take twenty-four hours, you probably won't get antsy until after those hours have passed. Let's say the banker gets back to you just four hours later; you will probably feel outright impressed. It's a wow experience because you didn't expect the information so quickly. Now imagine that the banker says initially, "I'll get back to you within two hours" but then takes three hours before calling you back. You are probably annoyed at the banker's failure to keep the promise. It isn't the actual length of the wait that matters. It's what you've been led to expect about the length of the wait, and whether that prediction turns out to be fact or fiction. The moral: in our services, we should be adjusting customer expectations (downward if necessary) so we can meet or exceed them.

*Institute scripts and script rehearsal so that staff members use magic—not tragic—words when communicating with patients about delays.* Develop and help people deliver in an authentic way *great* words of apology, explanation, empathy, and appreciation. See the figure on page 42 for sample scripts.

## A Wait-y Subject

Managing time—our own and our customers'—is not easy. Yet it's a compelling part of our patients' experience with us, and it's critical to patient satisfaction. The time is now to take the time.

## Scripts for Wait Lifting

### Adjust Expectations Immediately

**On the phone.** Suggest the length of time the visit will take so the customers can make arrangements. "I can give you an appointment time of ___. Because we can't predict exactly what help other patients will need before your visit, please expect to be here at least ___ hours, so you won't get anxious if you do need to wait."

**Upon arrival.** Offer the following to help patients accept the wait better:

- **Good intention:** "I want you to know how things work, so you'll know what to expect."
- **Facts:** "We take care of a lot of people. While we try to schedule so you don't have to wait, it's very hard. Sometimes, patients need more time than we predicted."
- **A good reason in the interest of the patient:** "We want to give every one of our patients all the help and information they came for, without rushing. Sometimes that causes others to wait."
- **Estimated wait:** "Today, my estimate is that you might be waiting about ___ minutes." Don't use the word "guess."
- **Thank you:** "I really appreciate your patience and understanding."
- **Offer comforts:** "Would you like _____ to help make the time go faster?"
- **Thank you:** "Again, thank you so much for your patience."

### Update the Patient and Family about Delays

- **Approach frequently:** At least every ten minutes, a staff person should walk over to the patient and family and give an update on the delay, letting them know they are not forgotten.
- **Provide a personal apology:** "Jimmy, Mrs. Hunt, I'm so sorry we haven't been able to take you yet. I want you to know we haven't forgotten about you!"
- **Explain the delay with the customer's perspective in mind:** For instance, "Other patients are taking longer than we predicted, and our care team wants to give each person the time needed."
- **Estimate the length of their wait:** "My estimate is that it will take another ___ or ___ minutes before we're ready for you. If that changes, I'll stop back and let you know." Don't say, "We have no idea when we'll be ready for you." Or "I can't promise anything." Or "Who knows when they'll be ready. It's a zoo today."

- **Empathize:** "I know it can be *hard* to wait when you aren't feeling well or you have other things you want to do."
- **Offer relief:** For instance, "Can I get you a magazine, or would you like some water?"
- **Apologize again and thank them:** Thank both the patient and family for their patience. "I'll be sure to let you know if there's a change."

Copyright ©2005 Wendy Leebov

• • •

# Additional Tools

## Tool 1
## SPEED MATTERS: A *WOW* PROTOCOL
## FOR HANDLING A DELAY

When patients and families are waiting, every minute feels like an hour. As people wait, impatience grows and tempers flare.

Because delays are such a significant source of patient dissatisfaction, adopt an organizationwide approach to dealing with delays. By standardizing the approach, managers can better engage staff in practicing and fine-tuning. When delays occur despite our best intentions, staff not only explain the delay but also communicate effectively their concern.

### A *Wow* Protocol for Handling Delays

Here's a widely applicable process for communicating with customers about delays. You can use it when you know there will be a delay and want to prepare the customer for what to expect. It can also be used if an unexpected delay has occurred.

- Address the customer in a calm manner.
- Acknowledge and apologize. Make it clear that you realize the customer has been kept waiting. Apologize even if it is not your fault: "I realize you've been waiting more than ___ minutes/hours, and I'm really sorry about that."

- State your positive intention. "I want to make sure the doctor sees you as soon as possible, and I want you to know what's going on that's causing a delay."
- Express empathy. Show that you understand the customer's feelings by saying, "I can imagine you feel impatient and concerned."
- Give the reason for the wait in a way that builds customer confidence. Say something reassuring: "We give each person the quality attention they deserve. Sometimes, this means that a visit will take longer than we'd planned. I can assure you we will give you that same quality of attention."
- Don't erode customer confidence or make your team look bad in their eyes. Don't say anything like this: "I'm sorry you're still waiting. We're short staffed. We're running ragged. One of our providers is out sick (or always late), and the doctor on call isn't here yet."
- Offer options for making the time go faster. "Would you like a cup of coffee or one of these magazines?" Or "Would you like to move to the area where you can see the aquarium or the TV?"
- Provide frequent updates. Revisit the customer at least once every ten minutes (for scheduled visits), half-hour (for unscheduled visits), or hour (for waiting family members) to acknowledge that you know they are still waiting, to tell them they are not forgotten, and to explain the continuing delay and give an estimate of how long the wait will be.
- Say thanks. Thank the person often for waiting, and make sure the caregiver who finally talks with the person thanks him or her again. Thank the person for waiting each and every time you approach to give an update.

Ask your marketing staff to produce a laminated card that spells out this best-practice approach. Then devote a month of e-mails and meeting agenda items to helping managers work with their staff to follow the card every day for a month. Help them take this *wow* approach from common knowledge to common practice.

## Tool 2
## SIX SCRIPTS FOR DEALING WITH LONG WAITS

Here are sample scripts for six situations in which delays play havoc with patient and family satisfaction. These situations also create embarrassment and stress for staff. Notice that best practices in dealing with unavoidable delays include showing empathy, stating your positive intent, explaining, making realistic time estimates, giving options, and expressing thanks.

| Situation | Words that Work |
|---|---|
| Waiting for discharge<br>• Tell the patient and family about the many steps in the discharge process. If most patients experience time lags between one step in the process and another, alert them in advance that this might occur, and tell them the reason in a positive way.<br>• Provide people with realistic time estimates and an overview of the process. In your explanations, it is better to overestimate how long the process will take and surprise them with a shorter time.<br>• Stop back and give the patient an update at least hourly. See if you can help him or her prepare or find a way to keep busy during the waiting time. | • Empathy: "I realize you're looking forward to going home tomorrow, and I can see that you're happy you're well enough to go."<br>• Positive intent: "I want to prepare you for the discharge process, so you'll know what you can expect tomorrow."<br>• Explanation:<br>—"I'm sorry to say that it takes several hours to do everything necessary before you can leave the building."<br>—"First, we'll wait for your doctor to check on you here one last time and sign the discharge order."<br>—"Since your doctor will be seeing many patients tomorrow, we can't tell you for sure how long he'll be with other patients before he gets to you."<br>—"Your doctor or nurse will (once again) go over the instructions with you, telling you things you and/or your family need to do at home to take care of you."<br>—"Your nurse or patient care associate will then help you get yourself and your things ready. This can take more than an hour."<br>—"Then, after all the right papers are signed and you're ready to go, we will arrange for an escort to help you to the door and ensure you have a ride home. Because we have many patients moving in and out, it can take a while before we can dedicate an escort to give you a safe ride to your car."<br>• Realistic time estimate: "You can see that there are several steps in the discharge process. That's why it will take up to ___ hours before you can actually leave."<br>• Thanks: "I really appreciate your patience." |
| 2. Waiting for pain medication | • Apology: "I'm so sorry you've been waiting for your pain medication."<br>• Explanation: "We had an emergency with another patient and got delayed."<br>• Empathy: "I realize it's awful to be in pain and not be able to relieve it."<br>• Positive intent: "I'm going to get your medication right away. I want you to be much more comfortable as soon as possible." |

(Continued on next page)

| Situation | Words that Work |
|---|---|
| 3. Waiting for the doctor | • Apology: "Mr./Ms. Jones, I'm so sorry about the wait. I realize you've been waiting ___ minutes already since the time of your appointment."<br>• Explanation: "The doctor is delayed" or "The doctor is taking longer than expected with another patient in need" or "The equipment we need for your test is being used by another physician."<br>• Positive intent: "I can assure you that you will receive the doctor's complete attention once she is ready to serve you."<br>• Realistic time estimate: "I think it will be as much as ___ minutes/hours before the doctor is ready. Would you like to use the phone to call and alert someone that you'll be longer than expected? Or can I get you something to make you more comfortable while you wait—a magazine, a cup of coffee?"<br>• Options: "If waiting for this appointment is making you late for something else, would you prefer to schedule an appointment for another time?" |
| 4. Waiting for diagnosis or care in the emergency department<br><br>(Did you know that care time is at most 19 percent of total time in the ED? That means wait time is 81 percent of total time!) | 1. Make sure the patient and friends and family have a written explanation of the care process, so that they're aware of the time-consuming things that happen in the ED. Help them understand how long they are likely to wait.<br>2. Explain duration. For instance, "I want you to know that you're likely to be here for at least ___ minutes/hours. I realize this may seem like a long time, but I'd like you to know why it will take so long."<br>3. Explain the reasons, such as:<br>　• "The doctor may be waiting for test results before being able to treat you."<br>　• "We need to see people with life-threatening problems before those who do not appear to have such serious problems."<br>　• "Because this is a teaching hospital, we have our physicians and residents talk with you and examine you, which also take time."<br>　• "There may be waits because of the tests the doctor thinks you need."<br>4. Ask what you can do to make their wait more comfortable. Show people where the phones and vending machines are. Give them the name of the person to ask for if they want an update before a caregiver is scheduled to give them one. |

(Continued on next page)

| Situation | Words that Work |
|-----------|-----------------|
| 5. Waiting for an inpatient room from ED or admissions | • Anticipation: Tell them what they can expect and why. "The process here has many steps in it. For that reason, it usually takes about (time estimate) before we can locate the right type of room for you and prepare that room by cleaning it and getting the right supplies delivered." <br>• Apology and empathy: "(Name), I'm sorry you're still waiting. I realize it's so frustrating to wait when you came here to see a doctor." <br>• Positive intent: "I assure you I will do all I can to take you in quickly." <br>• Explanation: "The problem is, for reasons I hope you'll understand, our policy is to take people in life-threatening situations ahead of people with problems that can wait. Also, because this is a teaching hospital, we have our physicians and residents talk with you and examine you, which also take time. There may also be waits because of the tests the doctor thinks you need. Then we need to find an appropriate room and go through the process of preparing it for you. This too can take a while as the patient in there before you might take more time than we expected to vacate the room." <br>• Realistic time estimate: "So getting you to a room is going to take a while—as long as _____." <br>• Options: "In the meantime, what can I do to make you more comfortable? Would you like to use a phone, read a magazine, or have some water?" <br>• Thanks: "Thanks for staying and waiting. I really appreciate your understanding." |
| 6. Waiting for a meal that's been delayed | • Empathy: "I'm so sorry that you haven't received your meal. I can imagine you're hungry." <br>• Explanation: "Apparently, when the delivery was made, you were out of the room." <br>• Positive intent: "I want to get a meal for you quickly." <br>• Actions: "I will immediately call food services to provide it. And I'll stop back in to let you know about how long it will take." <br>• Thanks: "I appreciate your patience." |

# Chapter 6

• • •

# Customer Rounds

*Have administrators visit patients so they
can learn what it's like to stay in your hospital.*

Making patient rounds isn't just for physicians. Chief executive officers and their executive team members can also make rounds. These visits with patients and their family members will provide executives with an understanding that can't be obtained from a survey. They also show staff members the hospital's mission in action, and the knowledge gained from making rounds can shape the organization's priorities.

Keep rounding simple by assigning four or five patient *room numbers* to each executive. Set the expectation that the executives should stop in the assigned rooms once a week to engage in conversation the patients and family members who are there. Because not everyone in those rooms will want to or be available to talk, expect each executive to successfully engage with two patients per week.

## A Practical Approach

You and your executives can take the following practical steps to ensure that the rounds are as helpful as possible.

Schedule a time each week when you will make your rounds. If you don't *schedule* rounds into your workday, it's unlikely that you'll make them.

When you arrive at a unit while making your rounds, find out the names of the patients assigned to your rooms before you enter. Knock before entering. If the door is closed, check with a nurse to see if a visit is feasible at this point.

## An Easy Introduction

Here are some simple ways to introduce yourself:

"Hello! My name is _____ and I am (position) here at _____
_____."

"Am I right that you are (patient's first and last name)?" (Wait for acknowledgment.)

If there are others in the room, say, "And I don't believe we've met" or "Are you family?" Acknowledge them, saying, "Nice meeting you," etc.

(Again looking at patient) "Well, Mr./Ms. _____ (and guests), I'm visiting a few of our patients because I'm interested in learning how our patients are feeling about their stay here. I'm wondering if you would mind talking with me for a few minutes." (If other people are in room, ask if the patient would prefer a time when no visitors are present.)

## Sample Questions

*Breaking the ice:* "How are things going for you so far in your stay here?"

*Comfort:* "While you're here, you're away from the comforts of home. How comfortable have we made you here?"

*Privacy:* "Patients have a lot of hospital staff coming in and out. How satisfied are you with their respect for your privacy?"

*Responsiveness:* "When you express a concern or ask for something, how satisfied have you been with your caregiver's response?"

*Communication:* "How well have the nurses explained things to you?"

*Recognition:* "You've met many of our staff members. Are there any people in particular who impressed you? Who? How? Would you mind if I thank them for their effort?"

*Advice:* "As a leader here, I want to make this hospital a great place for our patients. What can we do to make your stay here better?"

## A Gracious Goodbye

*Recap:* If you made promises, tell the patient what you will do to follow up.

*Remind about survey:* "Even though I was here today and asked you for your opinions, I hope you will fill out the survey you receive in the mail and return it to us. We read each and every survey and learn a lot from them."

*Say thanks:* Express appreciation for their time, opinions, and suggestions. And thank them for choosing your organization for their care.

*Wish the patient and family well:* "I hope all goes well for you in your remaining time here and that you do very well after you leave."

## Follow Up

*Provide on-the-spot feedback and follow-up:* If you hear a concern or complaint, follow up immediately by contacting the right staff member to ensure a timely response.

*Recognize stars:* Write a thank-you note to staff members who received praise from patients. Send the note to the person's *home*. Write, for example, "I had the pleasure of talking with a patient yesterday about their experience in our hospital. He mentioned you in particular as having impressed him with your care and service. Thank you so much for making this patient's day. I really appreciate the care and service you provide."

*Compare notes and pinpoint priorities:* Document what you hear on a personal digital assistant or paper. Spend five minutes at each executive team meeting sharing stories and reporting. Ask yourselves, "Given what we're hearing, are we doing the right things?" And, "How can we do better?"

By making patient rounds, you listen to the voice of your customers. You impress patients and their families and help them feel important. You exemplify your patient-centered mission, while showing support for and gaining credibility with staff. And as chief decision maker, you'll stay in touch and make decisions informed by the realities that patients and staff experience.

• • •

# Additional Tools

## Tool 1
## THE ROUNDING BLITZ:
## A SURE-FIRE WAY TO ENSURE ROUNDING

Has your team committed to rounding on patients and staff? And do they actually do the rounds regularly with enough people?

Most organizations committed to rounding leave it to individuals to schedule sufficient time for these rounds and to perform rounds when it is workable for them to do so. If people aren't doing the rounds when left to their own devices, dedicate a group meeting to then-and-there rounding:

1. At one team meeting a month, deploy people then and there to go and do one hour of rounds. At the end of the hour, reconvene and give each person a chance to share experiences. At the end, ask the group, "What conclusions do you draw?"
2. Discuss what actions need to be taken.
3. Clarify the date for the next rounding blitz.

## Tool 2
## COMPETITIVE ROUNDING

Here's another alternative to hounding about rounding. Do you find yourself having to prod and remind fellow executives and managers to fulfill their rounding responsibilities? Virtua Memorial Hospital in Burlington County, New Jersey, implemented this creative approach to promoting shared responsibility for completing rounds with both employees and patients.

• All leaders have to submit a log showing the rounds they've accomplished during a certain time period. Leaders are divided into high, medium, and low performers of rounds. Then they are assigned to six-person teams, each team consisting of two low-, two medium- and two high-performing rounders. If desired, each team can adopt a team name, such as its favorite football or baseball club. Or you can let each team invent its own name—which is considerably more fun and attention getting.

- There is then a period of months during which these teams compete in a rounding completion. It becomes the responsibility of the *team* to improve the performance of each individual on the team if they want a winning score or to avoid good-natured, but nevertheless public, embarrassment.
- Each week, scores for every team are posted, along with the list of each team's members. Only team members see the data about individuals on their team.
- What happens? Needless to say, peers help pressure each other to accomplish their rounds, so that no person is the weak link who drags down the team's score. Team members end up discussing what stands in the way and help each other. For instance, this system unearthed the fact that some people are very uncomfortable doing patient rounds. In that case, other team members have offered to do rounds together, to ease their co-worker's way.

## The Gist of It

1. Team up.
2. Keep score.
3. Post scores.
4. Chart each team's score over time.
5. Come up with a creative prize for every quarterly winner.
6. Keep the tone upbeat, not punitive. Use this system and the competitive spirit to make rounding happen.

# Chapter 7

• • •

# The Connective Tissue Issue

*Designed handoff communication
can help bridge the gap when patients
are transported between departments.*

It started when my sister couldn't breathe and was rushed to the emergency department (ED). After cardiac arrest, she was diagnosed with pneumonia and a heart attack. She was in the cardiac intensive care unit (ICU) for weeks—on a ventilator, unresponsive, with sepsis, minimal heart function, and what appeared to be the gradual shutdown of her bodily systems.

Thanks to phenomenal medical care, my sister's determination to hold her soon-to-be-born first grandchild, and lots of prayers by all of us who love her, the infections stemmed and my sister awakened. Over several months, she has slowly, painstakingly recuperated.

## Both Grateful and Appalled

Wow—the advances in medical care and the dedication of gifted caregivers saved my sister! I am grateful beyond words. But my sister has endured so many avoidable frustrations along the way.

Right now, I'm talking particularly about breakdowns in hospital *connective tissue*—transitions and handoffs—between levels of care, services, and members of the health care team.

My sister has been on a long trek across many levels of care for more than six months, from:

- Home to ED to intensive care
- Intensive care to a separately owned long-term acute care (LTAC) facility

- Room to room within the LTAC
- The LTAC to a tertiary care hospital's catheterization lab to a telemetry unit for follow-up on serious complications
- Cardiac care back to the LTAC
- The LTAC to a rehabilitation unit within a hospital
- Hopefully, in a few weeks, the rehab unit to home

Along the way, caregivers have said so many things that reflected breakdowns in the hospital connective tissue:

- "I'm just following orders. I don't know why this was ordered. And I'm not sure who the physician is who ordered it."
- "You're in a different service now. So you have a different doctor. I don't know yet who will be assigned to you. I'm sorry it has taken two days to see a doctor."
- "We need your bed, and we think you're ready to leave here. But we don't know if you'll meet the criteria of that other facility, because now you'll be treated as a new admission there even though you were there four days ago."
- "Who told you that? That isn't my understanding! I'll have to check!"
- "That must have been your day-shift nurse who said that. It's not my understanding."
- "That always happens here. One hand doesn't seem to know what the other hand is doing."

Not reassuring. With each move, there was a new admission process, different doctors, different staff, different setting, different criteria for admission and discharge, different care managers. With each move, there was a delayed start-up of food orders, confusion about who was her doctor, lack of communication between doctors resulting sometimes in no physician coverage at all or conflicting orders, new staff, shift changes, changes in medication, and more.

## We Need Process Improvement

Great handoffs are painstakingly *designed*. There are patient-flow consultants who can help when the disconnects are many, varied, and complex. But short of that, managers need to tackle and redesign disconnects between their service and others with which it interfaces. How about forming liaison teams? *Liaison teams* bring people together across department lines to smooth transitions and hand-offs. A liaison team is an *ongoing* team consisting of representatives of two—and always two—departments that interface routinely and whose customers will benefit from a good, solid bridge between the two departments. Some examples are pharmacy and nursing, nursing and maintenance/engineering, environmental services and nursing, transport and radiology, ED and computed tomography scan.

## Liaison Team Agenda

The liaison team needs to ask these questions:

- What handoffs are there between us?
- How can we streamline this handoff?
- What needs to happen so that this handoff is effective and satisfying for our customers?
- Should we develop "interdepartmental service contracts" that spell out what each department needs to do to hold up its end in serving a customer whose service cuts across both departments?

Or how about snag-specific process improvement teams? These teams should explore one or more of the following disconnects:

- Is there a time lag between admission and clarification about which physician will cover the patient and when?
- Does the nurse know the care plan, so he or she can implement it?
- Do patient belongings get lost between the emergency room and inpatient room?
- Does your phone system cut people off while they're on hold?
- When a patient goes from the reception area in outpatient services to an ancillary testing area, does his or her information go along?
- When the physician makes a medication change, does the change reach pharmacy and nursing in a timely fashion, so that there is no error?

- When a family member calls to send a message to a patient, does the patient receive it consistently?
- When the patient sees the doctor for a review of test results, has the doctor already received the results?
- When a new patient is about to be admitted, is environmental services alerted in time to prepare a clean room in a timely fashion?
- Is the receiving unit notified and ready with a greeter so the patient feels personally welcome and doesn't hear someone say, "Oh, no! Another patient!"?

We need to painstakingly design solutions.

## Instituting Key Words that Boost, Not Blame

Doctors blaming nurses. Nurses blaming doctors, pharmacy, radiology, and transport, and vice versa. And everybody blames administration or insurance companies. It doesn't help. It undermines patient and family confidence in their care, in their caregivers, and in the health care system.

### All One Team

When we present ourselves as part of a connected team of caregivers who respect and trust one another:

- We relieve patient and family anxiety.
- We make each other stronger.

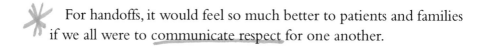 For handoffs, it would feel so much better to patients and families if we all were to communicate respect for one another.

Imagine a physician saying all of these things to the patient and family:

- **About the nurse and nursing team:** (Turning to nurse) "Thanks, Ms. Myers. (Then turning to patient) "Mrs. Morrow, Ms. Myers is terrific. I really enjoy working with her; you're lucky to have her."
- **About the doctor covering the next shift:** "I'll be leaving shortly, Mrs. Morrow. Dr. Marcus will be seeing you tonight. Before I go, I'll be sure to talk with Dr. Marcus about your day and your needs at this point. He's a great doctor. You'll be in good hands with him."
- **About the patient's attending physician:** "Mrs. Morrow, I see Dr. Richards is your physician. He is excellent. He's very good at explaining things and has a lot of empathy for his patients. You're in good hands with him."
- **About ancillary services:** "Mrs. Morrow, this afternoon you'll be going down to radiology for a CT scan. Radiology has state-of-the-art equipment and a very caring staff. They're expecting you and will take good care of you."

Now that my sister is off the ventilator and her tracheotomy has healed, thankfully, she has her voice back. Now that her voice is back, she is most certainly viewed as a very difficult patient. Having become hyper-vigilant because of the breakdowns, especially those during handoffs and transitions, she demands information, asks questions, expresses her impatience, and persists until she gets the clarity she needs. My sister is just trying to achieve a semblance of control and confidence as she moves from one disconnected step to another in her harrowing recovery process.

It would be so much easier for her and for the caring people who are tending to her if transitions during her care resembled the flow of water—smooth, continuous, and soothing, without barriers or obstructions. It's time to make patient flow from place to place, service to service, and person to person a smooth, continuous, and healing experience for patients and families.

• • •

# Additional Tools

## Tool 1
## QUESTIONS THAT HELP IDENTIFY OPPORTUNITIES
## TO STREAMLINE A HANDOFF PROCESS

Every time there's a handoff, there's time spent on it and the possibility of:

- A time lag, delay, and wasted time for the customer
- A delay and wasted time for staff
- Information falling through cracks
- Unforeseen circumstances that interrupt the flow
- Errors

To improve handoff processes, take the following steps: *design* them, and in so doing, *reduce the steps* and *reduce the number of different people* involved.

Ask these questions of yourself, your team, and other managers in areas that interface with yours:

1. How necessary is this handoff?
2. How can we have fewer people interfacing with the patient?
3. How can we diversify people's roles so they are doing more for the patient, instead of doing one thing and passing the patient to another specialist who does the next thing?
4. How necessary is each specific thing being asked of the patient? How can we streamline the process?
5. What can we do in advance to cut short the time needed from the patient once he or she arrives?
6. How can we make sure there's a person on the receiving end of a handoff—consistently?

## *Tool 2*
## THE WONDERFUL "PENGUIN POSTER" ABOUT HANDOFFS

### Did you know?

After the mother Emperor penguin lays a single egg, the father incubates the egg by holding it on top of his feet under folds of fat. For four months, he huddles together with other fathers and keeps the egg from freezing. When the egg hatches and the mother returns, the father transfers the chick from his feet to the feet of the mother Emperor penguin. They have to be very careful when they transfer the chick, because if it falls on the ground for more than a few minutes, it will die. . . .

### Lives are at stake.

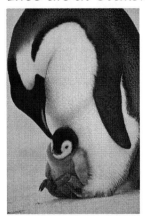

©2008 Frans Lanting/www.lanting.com

### Let's handoff our patients
### with painstaking care.

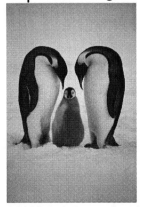

©2008 Frans Lanting/www.lanting.com

## *Tool 3*
# FIVE HANDOFF SCRIPTS

## Transporter—Transporting a patient

| Wow Behaviors | Wow Words |
|---|---|
| If you first touch base with staff, tell them why you're here and ask for any information about the patient that might help you. | • "Hi, I'm Jim Horne, and I'm here to escort Sara Roberts to x-ray."<br>• "Is there anything special I should know before I go for her?" |
| Enter the patient's room with respect. Always knock before entering. Announce yourself with your name and role. | "Hello, Ms. Roberts. I'm Jim Horne, your escort. May I come in?" |
| • Give an enthusiastic hello, as if this patient is the high point of your day.<br>• After you enter, make eye contact and give a big smile. Greet the patient warmly. Call him or her by name. Introduce yourself by your first and last name. Tell the patient your purpose. | • "Hello, Ms. Roberts. I'm Jim Horne, and I'm here to escort you to x-ray."<br>• Alternative: "Hello, Ms. Roberts. I'm Jim Horne, and I hear you're on your way to x-ray, and (pointing to wheelchair or stretcher), I'm here with your limousine (big smile)." |
| • Acknowledge family and visitors: face them and greet them warmly.<br>• Introduce yourself to them, too. | "Hello, I'm Jim Horne, and I'm going to help your loved one/dear one to x-ray." |
| Offer help: looking at and speaking directly to the patient, ask if he or she wants help onto the stretcher or wheelchair. | "Now, may I help you onto this wheelchair?" |
| Provide the patient with privacy and respect his or her dignity. Share your good intentions. | • "For your privacy, how about if I close this curtain while you get on the (stretcher or wheelchair)?"<br>• Also, how about if I cover you with this blanket/sheet for your privacy and comfort during your ride to x-ray?" |

*(Continued on next page)*

| Wow Behaviors | Wow Words |
|---|---|
| Offer last-minute help: Pause before leaving the room and ask if the patient needs anything else. | • "What else do you need before we're on our way?"<br><br>• If at discharge, "Would you like me to check for all your belongings before we're on our way?" Or, "How about if I check to make sure we have everything before we're on our way?" |
| Invite questions. Make it easy for the patient or family to ask them. If you don't know the answer, offer to go find someone who does. Make it easy for them to ask questions at any time. | • "Before we go, what questions do you have?"<br><br>• "Please let me know if you *do* have questions at any point, and I'll do my best to help." |
| As you walk through halls with the patient (and family):<br><br>• Ask the patient if he or she is in a condition to talk. If not, talk to him or her anyway. Don't proceed in silence, and don't proceed as if the patient isn't there.<br><br>• Act as a tour guide, giving constant updates about your progress (without expecting a response).<br><br>• Figure out a few routine comments or questions for this purpose. Ask a question; make an admiring comment.<br><br>• Say hello to people as you pass, whether or not you know them. Be a model of hospitality.<br><br>• Check often to make sure that the patient remains covered up and warm enough.<br><br>• Ask about the speed. | <br><br><br><br><br><br><br><br><br><br><br>• "Now we're passing our cafeteria and on our way to the radiology area. We just have to take a short elevator ride to the first floor," etc.<br><br>• "I hope you've had a good experience with us! Did any of my colleagues stand out for being wonderful? That's something I always like to know, so I can pass along that they are appreciated."<br><br>• Or, "Are you a sports fan, Ms. Roberts, or what do you enjoy, if you don't mind me asking?"<br><br><br>• "Is our speed okay, or are we going too fast?" |

*(Continued on next page)*

| Wow Behaviors | Wow Words |
|---|---|
| • Don't get into conversations with other staff unless you *include the patient.*<br><br>• If a visitor asks you for directions, turn to the patient and say: | • "Ms. Roberts, this is my good friend Bill. Bill is a _____ here. Bill, I'm Ms. Roberts' limousine service this morning!"<br><br>• "Ms. Roberts, I'd like to help this gentleman find his way. Would you mind?" |
| When you get where you're going, make a smooth, clear transition. Smoothly hand the patient off to another person before you leave. | "Ms. Roberts, here are we are at x-ray. I'll be going now to help another patient. I'll be sure my colleagues here know you've arrived. Please relax here, and my co-worker will take care of you shortly. You're in good hands here." |
| Clarify how the patient will be escorted back to the room when done, whether you or someone else will escort him or her. If not you, explain how this person will be notified. | "When you're finished here, a member of our team will call an escort to take you back to your room. I hope it's me, but it might not be." |
| Ask again if the patient needs anything before you leave. Listen to the response and act. | • "Is there anything I can do for you before I go?"<br><br>• If being discharged, add, "I hope you've had a good experience here with our team." Listen to the patient's response. |
| Provide a gracious goodbye. Still maintaining eye contact and smiling, thank and wish the patient well. | • "Thank you for coming to us for your care. I wish you the best and hope all goes well for you."<br><br>• If he or she says thank you, say "My pleasure!" |

## Physician—Arriving for daily visit, receives handoff from nurse at bedside

| Wow Behaviors | Wow Words |
|---|---|
| • Greet patient first. Address by preferred name. Smile, make eye contact. | "Good afternoon, Mrs. Smith." |
| • Greet nurse by name. Smile, make eye contact. | "Good afternoon, Helen." |
| Turn to the nurse without turning fully away from the patient. Make eye contact. | "So, is there anything I need to know from you about how Mrs. Smith is doing today?" |
| • Listen.<br>• Thank the nurse. | "Thank you, Helen. It looks like you've been taking wonderful care of Mrs. Smith. I'll take it from here." |
| • Turn back to patient.<br>• Smile and make eye contact. | "So, Mrs. Smith, tell me how you're feeling today." |

## Physician—Handing off patient to another physician

| Wow Behaviors | Wow Words |
|---|---|
| • Make eye contact, smile, use patient's name.<br>• Move to patient's level.<br>• Tell patient when you are leaving and what to expect.<br>• Let him or her know that you will check on his or her progress. | "I'll be leaving at 4, Mrs. Armstrong. It's now 2. I might not see you before I go, although I'll check on your progress with your nurse." |
| Let the patient know who will be taking over and that you will personally communicate patient's needs to next doctor. | "Starting at 4, Dr. Martin will take over your care. I'll make sure I tell Dr. Martin all about you." |
| Express confidence in your colleague. | "You'll be in good hands with Dr. Martin." |
| Open up for questions. (Be present and caring even though you're about to leave.) | "Do you have any questions or concerns before I go, Mrs. Armstrong?" |
| Say how you can be reached. | "Now, I want to be sure you know how you can reach me if you need to. . . ." |

## Person in Billing—Passing patient's phone complaint to person in patient care

| Wow Behaviors | Wow Words |
|---|---|
| • Apologize and thank the patient for the feedback. Tell him or her that you want to help.<br>• Address the patient by name. | "I'm so sorry you haven't received the quality of care you deserve, Mrs. Jones. But I'm glad you've brought this to our attention, and I want to help make it right." |
| Get the details and check back to make sure you've gotten it right. | "Now, I want to make sure that I understand the exact details of the situation. . . . Does that sound accurate?" |
| • Ask patient's permission to find out the appropriate patient care manager who can address the patient's complaint.<br>• Promise to call back the patient to give him or her the name of the patient care manager and explain next steps. | "I would like to call a colleague in patient care to find out who is the person who can best look into this for you. Would you mind if I make that call and then call you back? I'll do it right away." |
| • Update patient on name and how to contact colleague. | "Hello, Mrs. Jones. This is Helen Smith from _____ Hospital. Marna English will be happy to talk with you and follow up on your concern. She will call you today. How about if I give you Marna's name and number in case you want to reach her?" |
| Build up your colleague in the patient's mind. Express confidence that this colleague cares and will help. | "Marna is terrific, and she'll be sure to follow up." |
| Thank the patient for speaking up. | "Thanks again for speaking up, Mrs. Jones, so we can try make things right." |

# Person in Radiology—Transferring a misdirected phone call

| Wow Behaviors | Wow Words |
|---|---|
| • Keep in mind that the caller may have been transferred to several other offices before reaching yours. | • "May I have your name please?" |
| • If the caller reached you by mistake when trying to reach someone else in your organization, tell the caller which office he or she has reached and offer to transfer the call to the proper office. | • "I'm sorry, Mr. Mancini. This is Radiology, and you want Physical Therapy. I'll be glad to transfer your call to Physical Therapy. In case we get disconnected, or you get a busy signal, would you like to take down their direct number?" |
| • Take the time to understand what the caller needs and to figure out who he or she should actually be calling. | |
| • If you do not have the correct extension at your fingertips, take the time to look it up. | |
| • Be sure to give the caller the correct number for future reference and for use in case the transfer is disconnected. | • "Do you have a pencil handy? I'll be glad to wait." <br><br> • "Their number is 456-6666. Would you like me to repeat that for you?" |
| • When you transfer the call, stay on the line to make sure that you've connected the person with the correct department. | • "My pleasure." <br><br> • "Now please hold while I transfer your call, and thank you for calling." |

# Chapter 8

• • •

# Dealing with
# Difficult-for-Me People

*Showing compassion can greatly ease an otherwise
difficult patient-caregiver relationship.*

I feel sick at heart for the many wonderful, caring, and compassionate health care professionals who feel demoralized by patients, families, and colleagues they find difficult.

I admit, some people are truly difficult, but not nearly as many as
we might think. Having spent the better part of four months visiting
my sister in a variety of health care settings, I think many difficult
people are not inherently difficult. They are made to be difficult.

Thankfully, my sister just returned home, after receiving care, via
ambulance, emergency room, intensive care, critical care, radiology,
same-day surgery, long-term acute care, catheterization lab, cardiac
care, rehabilitation, primary care, and now home health. No one in
the emergency department or intensive care found my sister difficult.
I would hope not, since she was unconscious in those settings. But
after my feisty sister defied all odds and regained consciousness, she
gained a reputation as a difficult patient, and this reputation accom-
panied her to each new level of care.

## My Sister Difficult? No.

She was hooked up to a ventilator through her mouth and later her
neck, to a feeding tube, a central line, catheters, and to all kinds of mon-
itors, and she had gizmos on her legs to enhance circulation. On top
of that, she was placed in restraints for her own good so she wouldn't
dislodge any of these paraphernalia. Every orifice was invaded. For

another month, she could not move, let alone walk, breathe on her own, talk, or write. The call bell was her one-and-only communication device. And when she pushed that button, she wanted a response.

When she started to talk and asked, "When?" she was told, "Soon. You're not our only patient." When she asked, "Why not?" she was too often told, "It's against policy." When she asked, "How can I possibly do that?" she was told, "Toughen up, honey."

Time and again, she felt upset. A diplomat at heart, she complained nicely at first. But after a series of unresponsive indignities, she fought sleep because she was so afraid of what would happen if she took a rest from being vigilant on her own behalf. She became impatient and irritable, and she issued demands. What started as "Will you please ____?" turned into "I want it, and I want it now!" In her desperation, the time for politeness had ended because politeness was not working.

My sister felt desperate and out of control of her body and her life. That, combined with predictable intensive care unit psychosis, led her to behave in ways that some caregivers found maddeningly stressful.

It doesn't have to be that way. Without question, our health care colleagues mean well. The amazing clinical care my sister received takes my breath away. It saved her life. The people who choose health care professions care! They want what's best for people. And because they know they mean well, they feel affronted by patients and families who don't seem to appreciate that.

## Showing Our Caring

*If patients don't see caring, for them it isn't there.* The problem is not a lack of caring. The problem is a lack of showing it. We need to do and say things that make our caring and commitment to patients glaringly obvious.

The five-point plan that follows goes a long way toward reducing the number of (and angst created by) difficult-for-me patients.

### Reduce Difficult-for-Me Patients: A Five-Point Plan

1. Stop allowing bits of behavior that many patients find irritating.
2. Coach staff to express caring out loud—using words that reflect empathy.
3. Help staff stop taking demands, impatience, frustration, and pain as defiance or personal insults.
4. Institute regular processes that prevent desperation.
5. Build staff communication skills by focusing on the difficult situations that deplete their energy.

## Point 1: Stop Allowing Bits of Behavior that Many Patients Find Irritating

Some staff do things that predictably come back to haunt them. Here are a few examples.

| Irritating to Patients | Why? |
|---|---|
| Do the tasks; express no compassion | If you are exclusively task oriented and don't put your compassion into words, the patient thinks his or her pain, suffering, and discomfort are "ho-hum" for you. |
| Socialize outside their room | This creates the perception that you are goofing off, and when patients feel they need attention, this maddens them. |
| Wear strong colognes | Many people who are sick find perfumes and colognes nauseating. |
| Wear jangly jewelry | People who are sick are especially sensitive to clicks and clatters, squeaks and jangles. |
| Mosey in when responding to a call light | For patients, every minute is an hour. When they push the button and you don't display a sense of urgency, they doubt your caring. |
| Chewing gum, cracking gum | Many people find this nauseating to watch; when a caregiver is hovering over a patient, they don't tend to enjoy the sight, smell, or sound. |
| "Dear, honey, sweetie" | Some people don't mind, and caregivers certainly mean well, but many patients find it patronizing. |
| "Hold your horses" "You're not my only patient" "You'll have to be more patient" "We're short staffed" "Now what do you want?" | Patients and families feel dismissed and discounted when they hear these words. |

Engage teams in identifying the *hot button behaviors and words* in their roles with their customers. And make a pact to stop these from occurring.

## Point 2: Coach Staff to Express Caring Out Loud— Using Words that Reflect Empathy

Help your team communicate their caring and receive the gratitude and trust of patients and families. Help people speak the language of caring.

| Language that Shows Caring | Examples |
|---|---|
| Help staff acknowledge patients' feelings. | "This must be so hard for you." <br> "I'm so sorry about your pain." <br> "You seem discouraged." <br> "You seem tired." <br> "I can imagine this might feel scary." |
| Help staff use the words "for you" over and over. It forces staff to realize that what they're doing is for the patient. | "Let me open that for you." <br> "Let me close this curtain for you." <br> "Let me find your nurse for you." <br> "Let me find a more comfortable wheelchair for you." <br> "How about if I call your daughter for you?" |
| Help staff regularly state their positive intent. | "I want to make you comfortable." <br> "I want to keep you safe." <br> "I want to help you relax." <br> "I want to protect your privacy." <br> "I really want to help you." |
| Help staff express positive regard for patients and families, even for those who appear difficult. | "I admire your courage." <br> "I appreciate your patience." <br> "I really appreciate your devotion to your mom." <br> "Thank you so much for speaking up. It gives me the chance to correct this." <br> "I'm sorry it took so long. Thanks for understanding." |
| Help staff combine these language skills into powerful statements. | "I'm sorry you were frustrated. I'm here now, and I want to help!" |

I'm working with one inspirational leadership team on a house-wide strategy to strengthen the competency of communicating with empathy. We're encouraged to find that people can indeed learn to use the language of empathy.

### Point 3: Help Staff Stop Taking Demands, Impatience, Frustration, and Pain as Defiance or Personal Insults

Help staff alter their inner dialogue or "self-talk" so that they no longer take patient demands and impatience personally.

| If You Think This | Think This Instead |
|---|---|
| "Here she goes again! Now what!?" | "Let's see if I can build her trust, so she can relax."<br>"I have a chance to make a difference right now." |
| "I didn't deserve that outburst. Doesn't she know that I care?" | "She's sick and very upset. This outburst isn't about me." |

### Point 4: Institute Regular Processes that Prevent Desperation

Quick connecting and comfort rounds are two examples.

*Quick connecting.* When my sister was in a coma, I found it upsetting that people referred to her as "she" or "her." I decided to help care-givers see the person within. I covered the wall with family pictures and a big list of my sister's special gifts and enthusiasms. When care-givers entered the room, they couldn't help but read it; from then on, they called my sister Linda.

Why can't a nurse who is meeting a new patient devote three to five minutes to asking the patient and/or family a standard set of questions that help to find out about this person and their story? And why can't the nurse, with patient permission, post a few choice highlights on a white board so that co-workers also see this patient as a unique individual with a history, a life, passions, and hopes for the future?

This three- to five-minute quick-connecting process transforms the care relationship into a caring one. Caregivers see the patient as a person, not as "the heart," "the hip," or a stick figure in the bed.

*Comfort rounds.* We know patients will have to pee. We know they will get thirsty. They don't plan ahead for these things. Once they call for help, it's already urgent. Why wait until they call?

Comfort rounds are regular hourly rounds in which one staff member per unit (patient care associates, nursing assistants, and nurses all take turns) makes rounds and checks on the comfort *of every patient,* not just *his or her own patients.*

"Hi, Mrs. James. I'm in the neighborhood. Can I help you to the john?" Proactive, hourly comfort rounds reduce accidents, falls, messes, and cleanups, not to mention extreme patient frustration and indignity. Patients become less demanding and more trusting. They know they don't need to beg for attention to their most basic needs.

Then, to also prevent desperation and show caring, how about getting more insistent on the use of this simple script: "I want you to feel comfortable and secure. Before I go, is there anything else I can do for you?"

### Point 5: Build Staff Communication Skills by Focusing on the Difficult Situations that Deplete Their Energy

Sometimes health care professionals resist skill building on communication. "I already do this." "This is too basic." "This is insulting."

The good thing about difficult-for-me people and difficult situations is that people want to handle them better to reduce the stress caused by them. This presents a burning platform for training that meets with minimal if any resistance. Hold clinics on the difficult-for-me patient and nurture the trust-building and communication skills that drastically reduce the energy drain of difficult-for-me patients.

## The Punch Line

While *most* patients are not inherently difficult, many do act in ways that try the patience and compassion of health care professionals. The result: a downward spiral toward both patient and staff dissatisfaction.

We can change this unfortunate dynamic. We are not powerless. More often than not, by instituting process improvements that prevent patient distress and anxiety and by overtly communicating empathy and caring, our teams can win patient trust and cooperation. It's time to invest in developing our teams to achieve a new level of communication effectiveness that supports their caring work.

• • •

# Additional Tools

### Tool 1
## TACKLING THE BIG FIVE TOUGH SITUATIONS: A PLANNING WORKSHEET

Engage your team in identifying a short list of frequent and impactful difficult situations. Make these five situations your Difficult Situations Agenda and enlist pairs of staff members to address each and propose constructive approaches.

__Patient Situation?  __Co-worker Situation?
__Family Member Situation?  __Physician Situation?

| Difficult Situation | How Frequent? | Stress/ Anxiety Impact on Customer | Morale/ Stress Impact on Staff | Can We Prevent It or Lessen It? How? | Need Words for Handling It? | Priority |
|---|---|---|---|---|---|---|
|  |  |  |  |  |  |  |
|  |  |  |  |  |  |  |
|  |  |  |  |  |  |  |
|  |  |  |  |  |  |  |
|  |  |  |  |  |  |  |
|  |  |  |  |  |  |  |

### Tool 2
## HELP PEOPLE TAILOR KEY MESSAGE POINTS TO A SPECIFIC DIFFICULT SITUATION

### Meeting Agenda

1. Describe the meeting goal—to produce key communication message points for effectively handling a difficult situation to reduce the stress and anxiety for patients and staff.
2. State your personal commitment and enthusiasm for investing in plaguing, frequent difficult situations and figuring out what *great* looks and sounds like in those situations. Give a quick testimonial of a satisfying experience defusing a difficult situation with heart/empathy.

3. Explain how you'll work together on this—one difficult situation at a time.
4. Focus in on one situation. Develop key words and actions for handling that situation with caring and a more positive impact.
5. Engage people in trying out the approach several times. Then fine-tune it with them.
6. Engage your team in *making* reminder cards that identify the key elements in the approach.
7. Reach agreement on implementation and support.
8. Thank people for working together. Express appreciation and reiterate what everyone stands to gain from developing *great* responses to difficult situations.

## *Tool 3*
## MEETING PLAN TO IDENTIFY PROCESS IMPROVEMENTS THAT PREVENT DIFFICULT SITUATIONS

In a meeting or committee:

- Look back over your team's brainstorm of difficult situations. Focus on the situations that could, at least some of the time, be *prevented*. Group these situations together into categories. For example:
  —Wait time
  —Insurance
  —Complaints
  —Policy/patient education
  —Scheduling
  —Phone system
  —Access to providers
- Prioritize the categories by asking, "Process improvements in which of these areas would have the most impact on quality of service delivery and work-life here?"
- Pick the top three categories.
- Then, using the difficult situations as your guide, come up with ways to streamline and improve the processes in each category.
- Focus on improvements that will pack the most punch, ease the most anxiety, and eliminate the most irritations.
- Make a timeline and get commitments for follow through.
- Make sure you schedule frequent check-ins with the people involved so you can stay on a *proactive* and *successful* course to preventing difficult situations.

# Chapter 9

• • •

# The Gift of Customer Complaints

*Smart hospital leaders encourage criticism from patients because it helps them improve their service.*

Patients and other customers who go away mad tend to go away—to another provider if they have the option. Complaints are, therefore, a gift because they give you and your employees a second chance to make things right.

In the service sector, making things right for an unhappy customer is called *service recovery*. It means simply doing all you can to correct a wrong perceived by the customer—and doing it in such a way that satisfies the customer. Patients and other customers are impressed when you apologize, acknowledge their inconvenience or discomfort, try to solve the problem, provide alternatives, and keep your promises—and do so in a timely and courteous fashion.

Here's how you can institute and sustain effective service recovery throughout your organization:

*Articulate a welcoming, positive attitude toward complaints.* Help your managers see complaints as a golden opportunity to turn customers who are ready to leave into loyal ones. Sell your management team on effective service recovery. Help them believe that problems exist when patients say they do—anytime customers feel disappointed, dismayed, angry, or upset.

*Validate the time spent handling complaints.* Make it clear to managers that it is important to spend extra time with upset customers. Encourage managers to discuss backup, coverage, and buddy systems so that staff have alternatives when they need to spend time with a customer to address a complaint.

*Model excellent handling of complaints.* Teach by your own powerful example. Show managers that dissatisfied customers can end up grateful for your efforts to please them and meet their needs.

*Institute methods for inviting complaints.* Instead of relying on customers to speak up when they're disgruntled, use regular written surveys, install suggestion boxes, and teach staff to draw complaints from patients with simple questions such as, "How has your experience been today?"

*Equip all staff, not just your patient relations staff, with the skills they need to handle complaints effectively.* Sponsor organizationwide service recovery training. Expect managers to coach their employees on service recovery, providing practice for handling common complaints and giving on-the-spot help.

*Define appropriate responses, atonements, or compensatory actions.* With managers, set parameters within which employees may act to resolve complaints. Define the boundaries of their authority and clarify processes they should follow so they can solve customer problems rapidly. Make sure all managers address the following questions with their teams:

- How much freedom do I have to bend rules to satisfy a complaining customer?
- Under what circumstances is it OK for me to act without permission?
- How should I respond when I need money or special resources to satisfy the customer?
- Suppose a patient prefers a certain type of pillow for sleeping and we don't have it. Can I go out and buy one and be reimbursed? If so, what permission do I need?

- Suppose I need the cooperation of other people or departments to solve a problem. What channels do I need to go through to get that cooperation?
- I certainly want to follow through quickly for the sake of the customer, but at what point is the solution out of my realm?
- To whom do I go when I don't know what to do about a complaint?
- Who would be the correct person to contact to get the answers I need as quickly as possible?
- Under what circumstances am I required to tell my supervisor about a problem or complaint? Would that be only when I can't solve it myself?
- When am I expected to document a complaint, and how do I do that? Is there a special procedure?
- When is a written response to a complaint appropriate?
- Who writes the response, and what should such a response look like?
- If I hear the same complaints over and over from many people and the problem is beyond my ability or authority to solve or prevent, where can I take this problem so it will receive the attention it needs?

*Prevent complaints by improving service processes.* Expect managers to use a simple way to log complaints, even those that are resolved, so you can identify those "here we go again" problems. Then do what you can to prevent more complaints. It is a terrible waste of staff time and energy to maintain ineffective service processes that cause one customer after another to complain.

• • •

# Additional Tools

## Tool 1
## WRITING THE EFFECTIVE RESPONSE LETTER

### The Effective Response Letter

1.  Thank the person for speaking up. Express appreciation. For example, say, "Thank you so much for letting me know about your frustration with _____. I appreciate knowing what disappointed you, because we want to improve our services when there are problems." Summarize or paraphrase the specific complaint. If you are not specific, he or she will see your response as a standard form and feel disregarded.

2.  Apologize that the person's expectations were not met or that he or she felt frustrated, inconvenienced, or upset. You can apologize without admitting that the person is "right." For instance, "I'm so sorry we did not meet your expectations."

3.  Express empathy. For instance, "It sounds like you felt very frustrated and annoyed."

4.  Explain what you did or will do about the complaint.
    *   Did you investigate? If so, how? What did you discover? What did you do about it?
    *   Explain alternatives at this point, if any. Tell what you can do to fix the problem for this customer and what you can do to fix the problem for future customers. If you can't do anything to fix the problem for this customer, tell him or her what you will do to prevent the problem in the future.

5.  Express your hope that your letter helps, and thank the person again for caring enough to voice dissatisfaction. For instance, "Again, I appreciate you sharing your concern with me, as it gives me an opportunity to take action."

6.  Offer further contact, if the person seems to want it. For instance, "Please don't hesitate to call me if you would like to discuss this further. Also, if I can do anything to help you and your family in the future, please let me know."

### Tips
*   Use "personal" words (I, me, we, and you). If you use words like "our patients" or "management," it sounds to the reader like a stiff and impersonal response.
*   Make the tone conversational. Don't sound formal or bureaucratic.

## Tool 2
# REMINDER CARDS FOR THE BIG FIVE COMPLAINTS

Imagine how much better service recovery would be if each department or service had a standard way to handle its top five complaints in an excellent fashion.

Complaints tend to come in bunches. A particular department or service receives certain complaints repeatedly. When a complaint is frequent, the manager should engage the team in working out a standard process for handling the complaint (assuming it can't be prevented in the first place).

Spark a one-month organizationwide project in which you challenge all managers to work with their staff to produce *wow* language for dealing with their five most common customer complaints. Require them to turn in the results in the form of reminder cards—job aids for staff that remind them of effective language for dealing with one complaint at a time. Here's an example.

### Patient's Friend Wants an Update from the Nurse

| | |
|---|---|
| • Apologize for not being able to give this update. Explain the practice of updating only the patient's designated contact person for the sake of protecting the patient's privacy. | • "Ms. Harlan, I'm sorry I won't be able to directly give you an update about your loved one. I checked with the nurse and learned that the patient's contact person is _____. To protect patient privacy, our practice is to update that person only. That person can then communicate with others." |
| • Offer options, for instance, letting the patient and contact person know of the friend's interest, and taking a phone number. | • "What I can do for you is tell your loved one and the contact person that you want an update. I can give them your number, too." |
| • Make sure of follow through by you or nurse. | • "I really appreciate your understanding." |

Once all managers turn in the reminder cards for their service's "big five," pass them around, inviting other managers to comment and make suggestions. Also, hold a customer focus group to review the answers and see if customers have suggestions.

Create a pool of *wow* responses to unavoidable complaints.

Finally, require every manager to conduct staff rehearsals of the *wow* language scripts for their big five, and urge them to use these reminder cards when orienting new staff members.

# Chapter 10

• • •

# Working Better
# with Physicians

*The relationships you and your colleagues
have with physicians are pivotal.
These tactics and tips will help you
keep them in good shape.*

Most health care administrators operate within an intricate web of relationships with trustees, physicians, employees, payers, patients, the community, vendors, other health care organizations, and many more. As complex and tangled as this web can be, there is no doubt that relationships with physicians are central.

Your organization's position as *provider* of choice depends on these relationships. Also, the dynamics between your medical staff and your employees have a powerful effect on your organization's ability to be an *employer* of choice—to retain the talented staff who interact with physicians daily. Strained relationships with physicians fuel discontent and cause disillusioned administrators and frontline staff to jump ship in search of a less stressful environment.

## Effective Relationships with Physicians

Consider these six tactics that enable health care leaders to reap the benefits of productive and harmonious relationships with physicians.

## Six Key Leadership Tactics

1. **Build bridges. Manage up.**
   - Take deliberate steps to build a strong relationship, identifying common ground and cultivating a spirit of partnership.
   - Facilitate dialogue among physicians, nurses, and other key groups that need constructive working relationships and unity.
2. **Engage and listen.**
   - Encourage talk on policies, needs, programs, services, quality, safety, the practice environment, and much more.
   - Create a sense of inclusion; capitalize on their intellect, expertise, and ideas.
3. **Support the physician's business.**
   - Make it easy and convenient for physicians to care for their patients.
   - Provide appropriate support, such as marketing, public relations, patient service support, and the like.
4. **Communicate often and with courage.**
   - Check in with physicians frequently about their needs and how you and your team are doing.
   - Clarify what you want and expect.
   - Be direct with feedback.
   - Confront with tactful assertiveness when criticism is needed.
5. **Advocate for your team and organization.**
   - Facilitate mutual respect.
   - Address issues that threaten quality, the employee work climate, patient satisfaction, and the organization's financial health.
6. **Express and show appreciation.**
   - Personally say thanks often.
   - Institute a process that ensures frequent appreciation and positive regard.

# Six Tips for Enhancing Relationships

As is true in family as well as business networks, relationships need tending to become healthy, remain robust, and foster growth and a spirit of partnership. The following tips and tools can help in the process of tending important relationships with physicians.

### Tip 1: <u>Build Your Relationships with Physicians Proactively</u>

Initiate <u>conversations</u> that help you get to know the physician and allow you to help each physician achieve his or her goals and yours.

## Conversation on Goals

This conversation helps you support physicians as they pursue the challenges, interests, and goals important to them.

**<u>Talents</u>:** I want to help you build on your strengths here. What are some of the personal skills and assets that you bring to your work? What do you do well and want to build on?

**<u>Passion</u>:** I want to help you pursue your interests and do what energizes you. What are some things that you care about in or out of work? What gets you excited? What are you eager to learn more about? What do you want to accomplish?

**Experience:** I realize you bring a lot of experience here. What have you done or experienced in the past that could help our team or organization? What life experience do you have that you know could be valuable?

**<u>Challenges</u>:** I want to help you pursue challenges important to you. What are some opportunities you would like to explore? Are there areas you want to work on or develop?

**Future:** If there were no obstacles, nothing in your way, where would you like to see yourself in five years? What would you want to do right now, within your work here, to help you move in that direction?

## Conversation on Strengths

The more information you have about how an individual physician wants to be supported, the easier it will be for you to provide effective support. Here is a positive approach.

1.  Ask the physician to tell you about a success he or she had recently. "I want to know more about what is gratifying for you in your work. Please think about a time when you felt you were at your best. This could involve an experience with a patient, family, or colleague. The key is that you felt tremendous energy and confidence. Please tell me about that."

2. Ask him or her to tell the story of this success and talk about his or her behavior and feelings and what he or she takes pride in now about that experience. Probe:
   - What was the situation?
   - What did you do to be successful?
   - What was the outcome?
   - How did you feel about yourself and your work as a result of this experience?
   - Outside of yourself, what do you think contributed to your success? What supported you in the process?
3. What are some things I might do to help you have more successful experiences in this job?
4. Thank him or her for sharing this with you, mentioning a couple of specific things that particularly impressed you as you listened.

## Conversation on Style

This information helps you tailor your communications and expectations to the individual physician's preferred modes of operating. Interview each physician about his or her preferences, explaining that knowing this will help you provide effective support.

**Meetings:** How often do you like to meet?
**Communication:** What form of communication do you prefer? E-mail, weekly face-to-face meetings, phone calls, or a combination?
**Status reporting:** I would like you to keep me up to date on how you're doing and where you are in relation to any timelines or agreements we've established. How would you prefer to keep me up to date?
**Feedback:** How do you like to receive feedback? Written, in person, or both? How often?
**Autonomy:** How much autonomy or independence do you prefer? What do I need to do to respect that?

Create a schedule to interview one physician at a time (e.g., one per week, or a whole morning of appointments). You'll learn a lot you don't already know and have a better sense of possible directions you might pursue with each person. Also, your physician colleagues will feel your support.

## Tip 2: Engage Physicians in Creating Solutions

Address problems and needs together.

## The Engagement Model

| Process Step | Why This Step Is Important |
|---|---|
| 1. **Pinpoint goal, rationale, and your commitment.** | Physicians need to be clear on the goal, the rationale, and your determination to create results—with their help. |
| 2. **Establish common ground.** | This helps establish a partner mind-set. It says, "We both share a stake in this outcome and will benefit from it." |
| 3. **Invite physician perspective and ideas.** | Physicians need to feel heard and validated. They have their own perspectives, which can be helpful. They have ideas about alternative approaches, and they will be more likely to embrace a solution or change if they help shape it. |
| 4. **Express regard:** Respect, acknowledge, and build on the physician's ideas. | If you express your regard for his or her thinking, he or she will be more likely to listen to your reactions, support the solution, and allow you to guide him or her in new ways. |
| 5. **Reach and clarify agreements and responsibilities.** | Both of you need a shared understanding of what you decided and what's next in order to avoid misunderstandings. Physicians need to be clear on their commitments and responsibilities. |
| 6. **Express confidence and thanks.** | Physicians need to know you have faith in their abilities and support and that you appreciate their involvement and willingness to help. |

## Tip 3: When You Are Asking Something of a Physician, Communicate Clearly, Showing Him or Her Some Empathy

## Communicating a Change or Request

*For example: improving patient access by changing available appointment times*

| 1. Your main message | The problem, change, or expectation and what you are asking of the physician: <br><br> "We're learning from patient surveys and from complaint logs that our patients are clamoring for more evening and weekend hours. I'm asking for your help in creating a schedule that will work better for our patients and families." |
|---|---|
| 2. Why? Consequences and benefits | The consequences and benefits for patients, for the physician, for the team, for the organization, etc.: <br><br> "I know you want to do right by your patients. If we could offer more evening or weekend times, they would greatly appreciate it. They would be more likely to show up for appointments. And they would come in with a more positive outlook, making it easier to address their clinical needs. Also, both you and our hospital would be losing fewer patients to other providers." |
| 3. Pinch of empathy | Recognition that you are not taking the physician's time and energy lightly. Anticipate and acknowledge his or her concerns: <br><br> "I know you have your patients' best interests at heart and would like to satisfy them. And I realize that our evening and weekend hours may be a hardship for you and your family." |
| 4. Your personal commitment and request or expectation | Repeat your commitment and request: <br><br> "Still, I really want to work with you to see if there is any way we can expand our evening and/or weekend hours to make them more workable for patients and families. I'm determined to do all we can to make this happen." |
| 5. Appreciation and confidence | Express your thanks, positive outlook, and optimism: <br><br> "I appreciate your working with me on this. Together, I'm confident we can figure out some effective options." |

## Tip 4: Express Appreciation to the Physician— Frequently and Genuinely

An American Red Cross leader once said, "Reward is respect made visible." Make visible your respect for the valuable members of your team.

| Situation | Statement of Appreciation |
|---|---|
| The physician has waited a long time to discuss his or her resource needs. | "I realize we've kept you waiting for this. I really appreciate your patience." |
| You have been working alongside the physician quite intensely for a while, in patient care, in meetings, and elsewhere. | "We've been through a lot together today, and I just want you to know it's great to work with you." |
| The physician gives you a nice compliment as he or she introduces you to a family. | "I overheard your comment about me to your patient. I really appreciate your saying that. I know your vouching for me built their confidence." |
| The physician is very engaged with you in solving a systems problem. | "You know, Mark, I really appreciate your help on this. I know your ideas are going to lead to a better solution." |

Develop a recognition routine and hold yourself accountable. Create your own reminder system by programming a weekly appointment in your personal digital assistant or e-mail, a reminder message on your computer screen saver or in your voice mail. Supplement spontaneous recognition by dedicating a specific time when you'll make your appreciation known.

## Tip 5: Take the Physician's Pulse Regularly

Create a monthly check-in meeting with him or her and do a checkup. Invite questions and feelings, concerns and frustrations. Show your concern and empathy. Show respect and regard without judgment.

## Regular Check-in

1. How are things going for you lately?
2. What's working?
3. What isn't?
4. How can I help?

### Tip 6: Keep the Communication Flowing

Prevent the NETMA ("Nobody ever tells me anything") feeling by avoiding the following relationship killers:

- Going around the physician instead of dealing with him or her directly
- Making promises and then proceeding to break them
- Coming late to meetings—this indicates a disrespect for the physician's time and an exaggerated view of the importance of yours
- Turning your staff against a physician: Making insinuating comments or undermining remarks about him or her to staff so that they join you in feeling animosity toward him or her
- Expecting the physician to read your mind, instead of telling him or her what you want or need
- Doing a half-hearted or sloppy job when you commit to doing something for him or her
- Wasting a physician's time at meetings by not preparing
- Taking up a physician's time and disregarding his or her cues that say, "Not now"
- Expecting the physician's support but not supporting the physician
- Not returning phone calls
- Treating the physician with disrespect, calling it a "style thing" on your part and expecting him or her to adjust to your style
- Getting defensive when a physician gives you feedback you don't want to hear
- Complaining about a physician to your boss or his or her boss before you've done all you can to deal with him or her directly

In your relationships with physicians, think "fragile, handle with care." Patients, your organization, the physician, and your own stress level will reap the rewards.

• • •

# Additional Tools

## Tool 1
## THE GIMMICK THAT SPEAKS A THOUSAND WORDS

Physicians want to know that you respect their time. Many view your respect (or disrespect) for the time demands on them as a reflection of your respect (or disrespect) for them in general.

Unfortunately, you probably need some of their time so you can build your relationships, keep them in the loop, and involve them in the decisions and the future of your services.

### Use a Digital Timer to Show Your Respect

Adopt a practice of committing to a time limit for discussions and meetings. Approach physicians with a promise of a quick meeting:

- "Dr. Harried, I'm thinking about changing our clinic hours. I would like to talk with you about it for five minutes. When can you give me five minutes? I promise that's all it will take."
- "Dr. Newguy, as we begin our work together, I would like to learn about your likes and dislikes about how we communicate. May I have five minutes of your time at some point this week? I promise to take no more than five minutes."

Hold yourself accountable by using a digital timer that buzzes when your time is up. When the time comes, show up with your timer. You can find timers in hardware, office supply, and grocery stores; they cost $5 or less.

### Time Yourself at the Meeting

Start by reminding the physician of your promise to limit the length of the meeting. Then, in a showy fashion, set your timer. For example, "Dr. Swamped, I promised to take no more than five minutes of your precious time for this. I'm going to set my trusty timer to five minutes, so I'll be sure to stick to my promise."

Can you accomplish anything in such a short time? If you know you have only five minutes, you're much more likely to take a few minutes to plan ahead how you're going to milk those five minutes. By planning—by deciding in advance what exactly you want to know and say and by following your bulleted agenda—you can cover an amazing amount of ground quickly. With time pressure on you, you'll whiz through your issues and questions in a systematic and efficient fashion. Then, when the timer buzzes, you stop, no matter what. If the physician wants to continue the discussion, say, "I promised to take only five minutes. And our time is up. I'm happy to continue if you're sure you want to spend more time on this now."

By using a timer, you vividly demonstrate your respect for the physician's time while engaging him or her in important discussions.

## *Tool 2*
## THE NINETY-DAY PHYSICIAN CHECK-UP

Schedule a lunch or meeting with a physician after his or her first ninety days. Take stock. Use the ninety-day milestone as an opportunity to build your relationship and learn about the physician's perspective and needs.

### Ninety-Day Check-Up

- Give your appreciation. Say, "Congratulations on your first ninety days!"
- Ask questions:
  —"What's different from what you expected? What's different from what we led you to believe?"
  —"What are we doing well? What's working?"
  —"What's not working? What's not going well?"
  —"How is teamwork?"
  —"How is communication?"
  —"In your past experience as _____, what did you learn that might help us here? What systems or processes might benefit us?"
  —"What can we do to make your job better?"
- Issue compliments: "I see you _____, and it's having this positive effect _____."
- Follow up with a thank-you note to the physician's home.

**Process Tips**
- Probe by asking, "What happened specifically? What do you mean?" "You say you want better communication. What communication do you like? How often do you want it? How do you prefer getting it? Can you give me an example so I can better understand?"
- Take notes.

## Tool 3
# WHAT MAKES MATTERS WORSE
# WITH A COMPLAINING PHYSICIAN?

Here are seven ways to strain a relationship with a physician. Avoid them at all costs.

1. **Becoming defensive:** If we take complaints personally and say things like "I only work here" or "It's not my fault," we make matters worse. We need to keep calm; stay objective; and avoid judging, acting superior, or making excuses.

2. **Coldly citing "policy" as the reason we can't do what the physician wants:** "I'm sorry, but that's the way we do things here" or "It's our policy" infuriates physicians, because it seems we care more about protecting ourselves than serving their needs. We need to somehow give the physician at least one option in line with policy or find ways to bend rules when we know we're acting in the physician's and organization's best interest. And when the rule can't be bent, we can at least listen intently and, with great apology and sympathy, explain the reasons the rule benefits patients.

3. **Poor listening:** When you fail to really listen to a physician's complaints, when you interrupt him or her, act unconcerned, or minimize the complaints, you will increase the physician's hostility. Fix your attention on the physician. Nod, look concerned, and do all you can to absorb the feeling and content of their message so that he or she will feel listened to and so that you can respond effectively.

4. **Giving the run-around:** When we pass the buck, tell the physician to see someone else, or give an excuse that doesn't make sense, we further frustrate and alienate our physicians. If we need to shift the complaint to someone else, we should hand off the complaint ourselves, instead of making the physician do it.

5. **Showing "off-putting" nonverbal behavior:** When we look annoyed, fidget, appear impatient or rushed, avoid eye contact, or keep working on our paperwork, we put off physicians, making them feel unimportant and aggravating their dissatisfaction.

6. **Making false promises:** Sometimes in our fervor to make things right, we offer solutions we can't implement or promises we can't keep. It's better to stop at hearing the physician out and apologizing than it is to promise things that won't happen.

7. **Putting down our own organization:** We really look bad to physicians when we make remarks like, "We get complaints like this all the time" or "Sometimes I wonder what management thinks it's doing." The fact is, when a complaining physician is interacting with any one of us, we are our organization's ambassador of goodwill. If we condemn our organization, we make our organization and ourselves look bad and undermine the physician's confidence in us for the future.

# Chapter 11

• • •

# Less Turnover,
# Better Patient Care

*It's up to managers to clear the way
for employees so they can do their job:
caring for patients.*

In these days of disturbingly high turnover, many health care organizations devote substantial resources to employee recruitment. In the short run, it's a must, but it's often conducted at the expense of retention—like running water into the sink with the drain open.

High turnover is incredibly costly and stressful. It thrusts managers and staff into a frenzied cycle of recruitment, hiring, orientation, vacancies, recruitment, hiring, orientation, vacancies, recruitment.

High turnover is also devastating to service quality. The great people you have on staff overwork to fill gaps caused by vacancies. They run ragged and resent it. New people, once you find them, take time to develop collegial relationships with their teammates, the ease of communication that comes only with time, and organizational savvy about how to get things done. Vacancies cause jagged, inconsistent service.

What to do? Get serious about making your organization a great place to work for the people you already have and the new people you're about to get. Your success in serving patients depends on having a critical mass of high-performing people who are focused on their patients and their work, not on finding the escape hatch to their next job.

# Creating a Great Place to Work

While you can't *underpay* people if you want their satisfaction and loyalty, satisfaction is not about money. To be satisfied in their careers, employees:

- Want to be involved
- Need to be in the know
- Want to do a good job—to make a difference
- Itch for opportunities to learn and grow
- Expect to belong—to work in a supportive group
- Like to be treated as *individuals* with unique strengths and a life outside of work

Here is a five-step plan managers can use to keep their employees happy.

## Five-Point Tactical Plan

1. Remove barriers to providing top-notch care.
2. Keep your finger on your employees' pulse.
3. Sculpt the job; cater the job to the individual.
4. Hold yourself accountable for retention.
5. Communicate your regard with appreciation and thanks.

### Tactic 1: Remove Barriers to Providing Top-Notch Care

When there are resource constraints, employees feel like they're pushing boulders up mountains. When staff are met with "no, no, no" or "we're trying, but can't seem to move the system," they get demoralized and question whether the mission of the organization is really about patient care.

Adopt *barrier removal* as your number one great-place-to-work tactic, and tackle it with a sense of urgency. Become an advocate. Out of respect and support for your staff, make running interference your key role—be an indefatigable advocate with higher-ups and other departments for your staff so they can serve their patients/customers.

Invite staff to tell you the barriers they encounter and how they can be removed. Here's a meeting format that managers can use to engage their teams in eliminating barriers within their control.

## Staff Meeting to Identify Barriers

- Begin by discussing the barriers to delivering quality care and service. Let staff know that you are intent on eliminating obstacles. Build confidence by reminding people of barriers the group has overcome in the past.
- Ask the group to brainstorm specific everyday things that pose obstacles. As people brainstorm, write their responses on sticky notes, one barrier on each note.
- Stick the stickies on the wall, and ask the group to cluster them in categories such as policy issues, equipment issues, people issues, team relationship issues, communication issues, and systems issues.
- Once the group has clustered the ideas, divide the group into small teams and give each team one cluster to consider. The teams should sort the issues into these piles:
  —quick fixes: actions they can accomplish right away
  —breakthrough barriers: accomplishments that would make a big difference if they could only figure out how to achieve them
  —unpreventable barriers: those they might not be able to fix but can find ways to work around or minimize
- Have the teams present their findings to the whole group.
- Acknowledging their precious time, ask the teams to then look over the quick fixes to select those they can act on immediately and those they can handle down the line. Have them prioritize the quick fixes by considering the following questions:
  —Why do we feel this obstacle needs to be removed?
  —What will it take for us to do so?
  —What support, resources, or information will we need to help us?
  —What can our team expect from us, and by when?
- The teams then share their plans with the larger group, and the manager helps them organize the follow through.

Meetings like these engage everyone in easing job frustrations. But while teams can achieve some quick fixes themselves, many barriers to doing a good job extend beyond department walls. What do you do when nurses don't have enough linen delivered on time, or when no patient education materials are available to support the nurse's predischarge discussion with the patient and family, or when the food-warming system is inadequate and hostesses hear daily complaints about hot food arriving cold?

Rather than giving up, as so many managers do, you can use rapid cycle improvement approaches or bring in operational experts to redesign the workflow. These steps will help make it possible to serve patients efficiently and in ways that are manageable for staff. Employees want the conditions and resources to do a good job with patients. It's our job to shrink the obstacles that block their desire to help.

## Tactic 2: Keep Your Finger on Your Employees' Pulse

We have great people in health care—people with altruistic motives. So why do some managers appear surprised or start pointing a finger when employees adopt a routine approach to their job or, worse yet, head out the door? I think a large part of it has to do with a failure of managers to ask questions of and listen well to staff. In these hectic times, staff are running ragged, as are managers. With an out-of-touch manager, disillusioned staff members become more disillusioned, and their concerns escalate.

Managers need to create a *routine* way to take the employees' vital signs. While some organizations conduct employee satisfaction surveys, these surveys merely supplement; they don't replace the need for managers to take the pulse of their teams frequently and in a personal way. A short report card that managers can use appears on the next page.

You can circulate this report card at least once per quarter to find out how employees are feeling. Share the results openly in a meeting with the staff who took the survey. Thank people for their feedback. Show responsiveness to their perceptions by telling them what course corrections you plan (not want) to make. Invite their suggestions. Tell them you'll be asking them to fill this out again in three months so you can see how they're doing and how you're doing. By using a short homegrown survey like this, managers can gain valuable information about how their team members feel and can then take steps to enhance their work experience and relationships.

There are also powerful ways to obtain feedback using focus groups and individual interviews. Both help create *customized* employee satisfaction and retention initiatives that have greater power than generic solutions.

| My Manager . . . | Report Card | | | | |
|---|---|---|---|---|---|
| | A | B | C | D | F |
| 1. Has made an effort to get to know me and show respect for who I am. | | | | | |
| 2. Makes job expectations clear to me. | | | | | |
| 3. Communicates thoroughly and often so I feel in the loop. | | | | | |
| 4. Gives me honest, regular feedback about my performance. | | | | | |
| 5. Shows respect for my life outside of work. | | | | | |
| 6. Shows flexibility to help me manage the many facets of my life. | | | | | |
| 7. Encourages me to express my concerns and shows responsiveness. | | | | | |
| 8. Helps co-workers get along, so we have harmony within our team. | | | | | |
| 9. Helps me feel appreciated. | | | | | |
| 10. Advocates for what we need; removes barriers. | | | | | |
| 11. Finds ways to help us lighten up and have fun. | | | | | |
| 12. Provides learning opportunities; helps me grow. | | | | | |

My suggestions:

### Tactic 3: Sculpt the Job; Cater the Job to the Individual

*Job sculpting* involves using what we know about each employee to cus-tomize the job *to the individual,* building on their particular strengths, making their work schedules doable and their lives manageable. The age of generic solutions to people management is gone.

Some organizations are making *individual* work arrangements with caregivers. For instance, recruitment and retention "SWAT teams" work with one patient care unit at a time to address the issues that different individuals within that unit identify as interfering with their job satisfaction. These highly creative SWAT teams dig deep, creating unique contractual relationships with employees. For example, some employees arrange to take on an ambitious ten-month schedule with twelve-month pay so they can take summers off with their kids and still get paid. Some negotiate for conference attendance and addi-tional learning opportunities instead of certain other benefits. Some negotiate for tuition support for their children instead of themselves. Some negotiate for physical help for all patient lifting, so they can work despite back problems. While it is complicated to do job sculpt-ing to this degree, and it requires human resources guidance to stay within the law, imagine the talent and energy it unleashes for patient care and service.

### Tactic 4: Hold Yourself Accountable for Retention

Employees quit their managers more often than they quit their jobs or the organization. Embrace your responsibility for enhancing and sustaining employee satisfaction. Consider employee retention a key leadership competency in your job description and performance review, and develop your retention strategy and skills as part of your personal learning plan. Set a goal for reducing turnover.

### Tactic 5: Communicate Your Regard with Appreciation and Thanks

This strategy is nothing new, but it's too critical to avoid mention-ing. Managers need to generously give each employee *individualized* appreciation and thanks. If we want our employees to feel precious, we will call them by name. We will inquire about how they're doing.

We will notice and appreciate them. We will compliment them about specific things that they do well and specific ways they contribute. We will acknowledge big life events. We will take the time to write occasional thank-you notes and send them to home addresses so they're more likely to share them with their families. We will give this positive regard whether we're getting it from *our* bosses or not. Active, regular, specific, genuine employee recognition must become a job requirement of every manager.

## Dare We Put Employees on a Pedestal?

Health care really is about valuable human beings caring for vulnerable human beings. It is the work of the soul. Health care employees have always deserved to be admired and supported in their caring work. It is our job to create caring communities that help them flourish. They will feel gratified in their lives. Our patients will benefit by receiving the care and service they deserve. And your organization will be able to maintain a more experienced, harmonious, and stable team.

**• • •**

# Additional Tools

### Tool 1
## FIVE MINUTES THAT TRANSFORM
## THE PATIENT AND EMPLOYEE EXPERIENCE

Caregivers have become very, very, very task oriented. It's no wonder, given the pressures on them to document; serve patients in less time; deal with family members; and meet all safety, quality, HIPAA, and payer requirements. Many caregivers feel like they're running ragged. Patients and family members feel the divided nature of the caregiver's attention. While patients and families might appreciate all that the caregiver accomplishes on their behalf, they crave the kind of personal connection and undivided attention that build their trust and confidence.

## Make Personal Connections

What if we were to build into our care process with each patient a few minutes devoted to learning something about the patient that will help us see this patient as a person and treat him or her in a personal way? And what if we could share what we learn so our co-workers also would see the patient as a person?

Imagine if every caregiver followed a designed process—a routine—for making this quick personal connection with the patient and earning his or her trust right off the bat. The goal is to establish immediate rapport, to make the patient and family immediately feel your interest in them as people before getting down to the business at hand. The relationship forms, and it influences all interactions from then on.

## The Nurse's First Hello

- Put your stuff aside. Get clear on the patient's name. Knock.
- Approach the bedside. Sit. Tune in. Focus fully on the person.
- Make eye contact. Shake hands or touch the patient, if it seems appropriate.
- Introduce yourself and state your role.
- Ask the patient what he or she prefers to be called. Use that name.
- Tell the patient a little about your experience and your commitment to the patient.
- Before performing any tasks, get to know the person. Listen intently. Connect strongly. Be present. Say:
  —"Tell me, how are you feeling now?"
  —"Tell me a little about yourself."
  —"We know very good care means different things to different people. What does 'very good care' mean to you? What do we need to do for you to feel that you got very good care?"
  —Ask if you may write highlights on the whiteboard in the patient's room (for follow up).
- State your appreciation: "Thank you for talking with me. It will help me take good care of you." Touch the patient when it feels right.
- If family members are there, introduce yourself; make them feel important.

If the caregiver adds five minutes up front to build a trusting relationship with each patient, the trust that ensues saves time and gives both the patient and the caregiver a more gratifying experience.

Ask patient care managers to work with their teams to design, test, and fine-tune a standard process for building trust in the first five minutes. Then have them install this as the standard approach. They will find that this saves time; it does not require additional time. Why? Trust early on relaxes patients and families. They become less anxious about getting the caregiver's attention. They sound their call lights less. They relax in the good hands of the care team.

Care teams will find it satisfying for the patient *and* family and satisfying to them. Professionals, after all, enter health care because they want to help and support people in their time of need. With this approach, caregivers reconnect with the meaning in their work and feel much better about it.

## Tool 2
## RETENTION CONVERSATIONS

A great proportion of employee turnover occurs during the first year of employment. While hiring people who fit their jobs and the organization well diminishes turnover, it is also important to ensure a good start. With this tool, managers can identify early concerns and issues that, if left untended, could send employees to greener pastures.

The goals of the conversations are:

- To help employees feel the manager's interest about their welfare and to feel appreciated early on
- To inspire employees to become even more effective and take steps to achieve a greater sense of contribution and satisfaction from their work
- To nip employment issues in the bud and retain the employee

Here is a sample opening: "Helen, I want to schedule some time with you to learn how your experience has been here so far. I want you to be happy here, and I want you to stay. Can we schedule a time for that conversation?"

In that conversation:

- State your intention up front: to help the employee find satisfaction in the job so that he or she chooses to stay.
- Start with very specific appreciation. What do you see as this person's strengths and contributions already? Express heartfelt appreciation.

- Take stock: Find out how they've been feeling in the job. Ask:
  —"How has it met your expectations?"
  —"How has it failed to meet your expectations?"
  —"Any surprises in it (and their consequences)?"
  —"What would need to happen here for you to find the job satisfying? What would have to happen to encourage you to stay?"
- Describe the big picture—where the organization is going. Bring this person into the loop on strategic direction. Say that you see him or her as an important contributor to this.
- Find out how you can support the employee's development and performance.
- Thank the employee again for all he or she does.
- Repeat your bottom line: "I hope you will stay and be a key player in our future. Please let me know if and when you have concerns that are interfering with your satisfaction at work."
- Once again, state your appreciation: Thank the employee.

# Chapter 12

• • •

# How to Create a Patient Satisfaction Epidemic

*Engage not only managers but also frontline staff to inspire better performance and create a groundswell of change.*

Many health care organizations start off culture change strategies with a bang, then allow them to fade quietly into disillusionment. Multiple priorities and battle fatigue make it difficult to stay focused, persist, and strengthen strategic effort. I've seen this time and again with service excellence and patient satisfaction strategies.

## Square Pegs in Round Holes

Effective follow through depends on managers to lead the charge, engaging their teams to redesign behavior and master skills. Yet, even with substantial training and coaching, many managers prove unable or unwilling to inspire their teams. Maybe they aren't focused on it, or they aren't inspirational by nature, or maybe performance management is not their forte and they don't devote time and skill to it.

You might be thinking, "These managers must be held accountable. If they can't lead the charge, then they need to leave the organization." That's easy to say, but usually, for a whole host of reasons, executives hang on to managers who just don't do what's needed. Haranguing executives about this hasn't worked.

Daring to be controversial, I'm suggesting that we need to find creative approaches to *spread*—to earn the gradual involvement of everyone until the change strategy has permeated the organization. We need to expand the internal capability of skilled people who champion the cause and can apply nuts-and-bolts skills to redesign key service interactions, rehearse and master improved approaches, and cement new habits.

I want to be realistic. When managers fail to inspire, this approach is a way to keep your patient satisfaction strategy moving instead of letting it die on the vine.

## Mobilize Squads of Employee Champions

I hope you read the terrific book *The Tipping Point* by Malcolm Gladwell (Back Bay Books, 2002). Gladwell shares evidence that significant culture changes reach a tipping point not as a result of a linear, planned change process but because a critical mass of people with certain predilections all apply their energies, even unconsciously, to bringing about the change. Their natural style, which they can't resist because that's who they are, pushes the change they want over its tipping point, causing it first to spread like an epidemic and then to stick.

Gladwell says that a critical mass of three kinds of people who may not even know or communicate with one another lead a culture change to its tipping point: connectors, information mavens, and promoters.

*Connectors* tend to be extroverts. They network with others constantly and greatly enjoy connecting people to each other.

*Information mavens* are resourceful people who love know-how. They're always engaged in learning something new, and they collect and savor concrete tools for accomplishing things important to them.

*Promoters* are people who can sell anybody on anything. They have contagious enthusiasm for what they believe in, they know how to sell the benefits, and they inspire others to buy in.

Instead of labored strategies to deepen patient satisfaction, how about a tipping point approach? Why not identify connectors, information mavens, and promoters from all levels of your organization—especially from frontline staff—and focus them all on the same goal: enhancing the patient experience? Why not take the principle Gladwell identified as an *organic* approach to change and employ a *deliberate* strategy to trigger that organic approach when it isn't happening by itself? This might sound like a paradox, but I've found that it works.

## Build and Set Loose a Squad of Peer Coaches

How can you take on this deliberate strategy to trigger a powerful, organic change process? By developing and proliferating squads of employees whom you develop as *peer coaches*. Develop them to do three things:

- Strengthen their role as informal opinion leaders. Heighten their passion for enhancing the patient experience so they cannot resist making their views contagious.
- Equip them to design good-to-great performance.
- Train them as performance coaches for individuals and job-specific groups of peers.

## Suggested Steps

1. Ask around and identify your organization's connectors, information mavens, and promoters.
2. Invite them to be part of a pilot boot camp for peer coaches. Tell them they have been identified as opinion leaders. Explain that you want to enlist their help in enhancing the patient experience in ways that will be fun and enriching to them.
3. Engage them in an intensive off-site boot camp experience.
4. Convene managers and orient them to the boot camp process. Have peer coaches talk about their training and their commitment as well as what they think they can do to help managers engage employees and improve performance.
5. When others in the organization ask why they weren't invited, tell them that the first round was a pilot, and that now you would be glad to include them in the next group.

Set up one boot camp after another to mobilize increasing numbers of the amazing and committed people you have in your organization.

## Introducing Peer Coaches

Here is a sample of a promotional flier given to managers to explain how peer coaches can be of help to them and their teams.

*Peer Coaches Available!*

## Managers, here's what peer coaches can do for you:

1. Peer coaches will be role models. They will demonstrate service excellence skills with patients, families, and other customers. They will make exceptional service their standard practice.
2. Peer coaches will promote a culture of service excellence. They will express their commitment and share personal testimonials about how this process is affecting them, how it is connecting with their personal hopes and vision for their work. They will do their best to address other people's resistance with courage, tact, and compassion.
3. Peer coaches will provide skill coaching in a supportive, helpful, and nonthreatening way. They will help people in their own and/or other departments with:
   - Key words design
   - Group rehearsals
   - Individual coaching

The peer coaches will *not*:

- Communicate performance expectations
- Discuss the timeline whereby performance changes must be made
- Confront low performers about their performance problems
- Manage ongoing performance
- Hold people accountable

These continue to be the manager's responsibilities.

## The manager's responsibilities:

- Prepare a Peer Coach Request Form (included).
- Identify the people who will receive peer coaching.
- Set up meeting times and places.
- Invite people to attend; communicate the purpose to them.
- Get people to show up.
- Thank the people who participated.
- Work with people afterward. Follow up; find out what happened. Proceed with performance management (e.g., install key words as expectations, communicate expectations, recognize improvements, and hold people accountable).
- Thank the peer coach for his or her help.

Below is a memo that can accompany the promotional flier. It gives managers more details on how peer coaches can help and what managers need to do in working with peer coaches.

## Peer Coach Service Options

| Service Option | Manager's Duties Beforehand | Manager's Duties Afterward |
|---|---|---|
| Designing job-specific key words with groups | • Submit Peer Coach Request Form.<br>• Attach existing key words (to be improved).<br>• Set up meeting; prepare attendees in upbeat way. | • Thank people for participating.<br>• Send personal thank-you note to coach.<br>• Review results and fine-tune.<br>• Talk with people about expectations.<br>• Manage performance.<br>• Hold people accountable. |
| Conducting group rehearsals | • Submit Peer Coach Request Form, attaching key words that people are supposed to rehearse.<br>• Set up the meeting.<br>• Prepare those involved. | • Thank group for participating.<br>• Send personal thank-you note to coach.<br>• Talk with people about expectations.<br>• Manage performance.<br>• Recognize improvements.<br>• Hold people accountable. |
| Coaching with individuals | • Submit Peer Coach Request (without name of person).<br>• Describe your goals for coaching.<br>• Provide information to help peer coach.<br>• Attach relevant key words.<br>• Prepare the individual receiving the coaching: "I've asked _____ to help you strengthen your performance. Here's why. . . ."<br>• Reassure that the coaching will be *confidential* and of a supportive nature.<br>• Reiterate your hopes and your confidence. | • Thank employee for participating.<br>• Send personal thank-you note to coach.<br>• Review results.<br>• Communicate your expectations.<br>• Manage person's performance.<br>• Recognize improvements.<br>• Hold person accountable. |

*(Continued on next page)*

| Service Option | Manager's Duties Beforehand | Manager's Duties Afterward |
|---|---|---|
| Orienting new people | • Submit Peer Coach Request Form<br>• Describe your goals for coaching.<br>• Provide information to help peer coach.<br>• Attach relevant key words.<br>• Prepare the individual receiving the coaching: "I've asked _____ to talk with you about our service excellence process and review with you how you can be a key contributor."<br>• Reassure that the coaching will be confidential and of a supportive nature.<br>• Reiterate your hopes and your confidence. | • Thank employee for participating.<br>• Send personal thank-you note to coach.<br>• Talk with new person about your expectations.<br>• Manage person's performance.<br>• Appreciate effective performance.<br>• Hold person accountable. |

Here is a sample of a Peer Coach Request Form that compels managers to think through their goals and provide the peer coach with relevant resources that already exist.

---

**Peer Coach Request Form**       Date _____

Manager's name _____ Department _____

For scheduling/questions: Phone _____ E-mail _____

Your goal for peer coach:


Background facts:


Number of participants _____

How were they selected? _____

| Service Option | Required Attachments | Attached? |
|---|---|---|
| Designing job-specific key words with groups | Existing key words, if any | |
| Conducting group rehearsals | Key words to be rehearsed | |
| Coaching with individuals | Key words to be rehearsed | |
| Orienting new people to caring culture and job-specific key words | Key words to be reviewed | |

I agree to the following:
- I will prepare all employees who will be coached so that they know why they are involved.
- I will make it clear that they will be helped by peers who will keep specifics confidential and serve as a guide/coach.
- I will make it clear that the coach is not responsible for implementing the results; I am.

Signed,


_____
Manager

---

# A Quickie Tool Kit

Here are some tools that should make the process much clearer.

## Peer Coach Boot Camp: Sample Agenda

### Day One

1. **Introduction/overview**
   - Kick off the boot camp, explaining why it's necessary; outline hopes.
   - Give goals and roles for peer coaches.
   - Explain *Tipping Point* and the power of connectors, information mavens, and promoters. Have people do some self-analysis to share their strengths.
   - Present three main roles for peer coaches (providing inspiration and serving as a powerful role model as well as a performance coach with peers).

2. **Becoming an inspiration**
   - Have attendees share personal stories about their commitment to health care and high points in helping.
   - Let them try out on each other an inspirational, personal statement of their commitment to elevating the patient experience.

3. **Becoming a powerful role model**
   - Help people realize the vast difference between inoffensive behavior and amazing, impressive, compassionate behavior.
   - Have small groups do bad, good, and great skits—stretching from awful to wonderful.

4. **Becoming a peer performance coach**
   - Explain the service options and process for getting assignments from managers.
   - Explore a set of tools peer coaches can use (meeting formats, rehearsal exercises, tips for script development, and more).

5. **Developing coaching skills**
   - Focus on the skills involved in being an effective coach, paying special attention to being an empathetic listener, asking instead of telling, giving constructive feedback, and the like.

6. **Inspire others**
   - Design and deliver "elevator speeches"—quick personal rationales and statements of commitment to improving the patient experience.

**Homework between Sessions**

- Sharpen your own skills to be an effective role model. Use your *great* greetings, handoffs, and goodbyes in your work.
- Watch for others' examples of great greetings, handoffs, and goodbyes.
- Find an opportunity to advocate for service excellence.
- Tell someone with whom you work about your peer coaching training. Say what's exciting.
- Come to Day Two prepared to share your experience.

## Day Two (a month later)

Share homework experiences.

**Key words design:** Demonstrate how peer coaches can lead individuals and teams in identifying best practices that result in consistently positive perceptions by patients and other customers. Best practices include scripts or impressive words for key interactions, such as greetings, transferring a call, making a handoff to a co-worker, handling a recurrent complaint.

- Discuss how to run performance rehearsals.
- Outline characteristics of a helping/coaching relationship.

**Review the tools:** What are we saying peer coaches can do?

- Practice handling co-worker resistance: some co-workers, when assigned to a peer coach, might feel defensive, annoyed, insulted, or resentful and might say things that make it difficult for the peer coach to stay focused on the goal.

**Strength bombardment:** To build this group of coaches as a team, here is a great exercise to help them appreciate each other. Ask peer coaches to identify one or two strengths they see in each of the other peer coaches—strengths they think will make that person effective and inspiring as a peer coach. Then the whole group takes turns delivering positive regard to each peer coach.

**Management briefing at end of day:** All managers arrive, and peer coaches orient them to ways they can help them.

**Follow-up**

- Have periodic check-in meetings with peer coaches, swapping stories of success and giving mutual support.
- In management meetings, feature managers who have benefited from peer coaches and spread the word.

## Create a Healthy Epidemic

Get it going and hope that other employees will ask, "Why wasn't I chosen?" Then develop another group of peer coaches, and another, and another. Imagine growing numbers of employees (not only managers) who are all inspired, mobilized, helping, and leading the way.

Developing a squad of peer coaches can help you deepen and expand your change strategy by engaging more and more people who will eventually move your hoped-for change to its tipping point—when you see it really take hold.

• • •

# Additional Tools

### Tool 1
### PEER COACH ASSIGNMENTS

Use these ideas as homework between boot camp sessions to engage people actively in the process and keep the energy flowing.

### Role Model
- Use your own *great* practices/scripts. At our next meeting, we'll share stories and results.
- Listen to others for examples of *great* language. At our next meeting, we'll find out what people are hearing.

### Advocate
- Find an opportunity to advocate for service excellence. Come back ready to talk about what you did that worked and what questions you have about advocating successfully.
- Tell a co-worker about your peer coaching training. Share your excitement.

### Scout
- Identify three missed opportunities—situations where you see a colleague miss a chance to *wow* a customer. When we reconvene, we'll use these situations to practice giving courageous feedback in a respectful way.
- Give the gift of ta-daahs. As you go about your work, make an effort to notice five situations when you think a co-worker performed in a *wow* fashion. Give the person a big ta-daah and specific feedback about the behavior and its positive impact from your viewpoint.

## *Tool 2*
## MANAGER'S INVITATION TO A PEER COACH

---

**Manager's Invitation to a Peer Coach**

My Name:

My Phone:

My E-mail:

I would like feedback about our team's _____.

I would like someone to:

____ Make "mystery phone calls" to my department

____ Come in person and observe our patient flow from a customer viewpoint

____ Come in person and discreetly observe our customers receiving service

____ Accompany patient and/or family member(s) through our service

____ Call me to discuss other ways we might benefit from your service-oriented viewpoint.

Please e-mail or call me if you're willing to help.

Thanks!

---

## *Tool 3*
## HOW TO HOLD KEY WORD/SCRIPT REHEARSALS WITH PEERS

Peer coaches can work with small teams of staff, helping them to practice their job-specific key words.

1. Explain purpose: to practice and get *great* at key words/scripts, so people can perform these skillfully and with ease in their daily work.
2. In a staff meeting or work team, divide staff into threes, with each trio designating a person A, person B, and person C. Then complete the following steps:
   - Person A chooses one of their key scripts and sets the scene. Person A practices his or her script on person B. Then B and C give feedback on what was effective and on how A's approach could become more effective.

- Then persons B and C take turns, each practicing and getting feedback before moving on.
- If time allows, repeat this process for *great* approaches to other situations.

3. At the end, convene the group and invite people to talk about what was hard, what was easy, and what advice they gave to others. This will maximize everyone's effectiveness.

4. Set date for a check-up meeting.

# Appendix

• • •

# Additional Resources
# for Health Care Leaders

## On Leadership

Ashkenas, R., Ulrich, D., Jick, T., and Kerr, S., *The Boundaryless Organization: Breaking the Chains of Organizational Structure* (San Francisco: Jossey-Bass, 2002).

Boyatzis, R., and McKee, A., *Resonant Leadership: Renewing Yourself and Connecting with Others through Mindfulness, Hope, and Compassion* (Cambridge, MA: Harvard Business School Press, 2005).

Collins, J., *Good to Great: Why Some Companies Make the Leap . . . And Others Don't* (New York: Collins, 2001).

Covey, S., *The 8th Habit Personal Workbook: Strategies to Take You from Effectiveness to Greatness* (New York: Free Press, 2006).

Gladwell, M., *The Tipping Point: How Little Things Can Make a Big Difference* (New York: Back Bay Books, 2002).

Goleman, D., *Primal Leadership: Learning to Lead with Emotional Intelligence* (Cambridge, MA: Harvard Business School Press, 2002).

Henly, K., "Detoxifying a Toxic Leader," *Innovative Leader* (June 2003).

Hunt, J., and Weintraub, J., *The Coaching Manager: Developing Top Talent in Business* (Thousand Oaks, CA: Sage Publications, 2002).

Kotter, J., *Leading Change* (Cambridge, MA: Harvard Business School Press, 1996).

Kouzes, J., and Posner, B., *A Leader's Legacy* (San Francisco: Jossey-Bass, 2006).

Leebov, W., and Scott, G., *Health Care Managers in Transition: Shifting Roles and Changing Organizations* (San Francisco: Jossey-Bass, 1990).

Leebov, W., and Scott, G., *The Indispensable Health Care Manager: Success Strategies for a Changing Environment* (San Francisco: Jossey-Bass, 2002).

Sanborn, M., *The Fred Factor: How Passion in Your Work and Life Can Turn the Ordinary into the Extraordinary* (New York: Currency, 2004).

Whicker, M., *Toxic Leaders: When Organizations Go Bad* (Westport, CT: Quorum Books, 1996).

## On Time and Priority Management

Bossidy, L., Charam, R., and Burck, C., *Execution: The Discipline of Getting Things Done* (New York: Crown Business, 2002).

Covey, S., Merrill, A. R., and Merrill, R. R., *First Things First: To Live, to Love, to Learn, to Leave a Legacy* (New York: Free Press, 1996).

Linenberger, M., *Total Workday Control Using Microsoft Outlook: The Eight Best Practices of Task and E-Mail Management* (San Ramon, CA: New Academy Publishers, 2006).

Morgenstern, J., *Time Management from the Inside Out: The Foolproof System for Taking Control of Your Schedule—and Your Life* (New York: Owl Books, 2004).

Neiman, R., *Execution Plain and Simple: Twelve Steps to Achieving Any Goal On Time and On Budget* (New York: McGraw-Hill, 2004).

## On Leading Change

Conger, J., Spreitzer, G., and Lawler, E., *The Leader's Change Handbook: An Essential Guide to Setting Direction and Taking Action* (San Francisco: Jossey-Bass, 1998).

Gandossy, R., Verma, N., and Tucker, E., *Workforce Wake-up Call: Your Workforce Is Changing. Are You?* (New York: John Wiley, 2006).

Schmeling, W., *Facing Change in Health Care: Learning Faster in Tough Times* (Chicago: AHA Press, 1996).

Schwartz, P., *The Art of the Long View: Planning for the Future in an Uncertain World* (New York: Currency, 1996).

Seligman, M., *Learned Optimism: How to Change Your Mind and Your Life* (New York: Vintage, 2006).

Senge, P., Kleiner, A., Roberts, C., Ross, R., and Smith, B., *The Fifth Discipline Fieldbook* (New York: Currency, 1994).

Senge, P., Kleiner, A., Roberts, C., and Roth, G., *The Dance of Change: The Challenges to Sustaining Momentum in Learning Organizations* (New York: Currency, 1999).

Wheatley, M., *Turning to One Another: Simple Conversations to Restore Hope to the Future* (San Francisco: Berrett-Koehler, 2002).

## On Relationships and Communication

Aguilar, L., "OUCH! That Stereotype Hurts," a powerful video on how to confront hurtful co-worker comments (available at www.learncom.com/index.do).

Bartholomew, K., *Ending Nurse-to-Nurse Hostility: Why Nurses Eat Their Young and Each Other* (Marblehead, MA: HCPro, 2006).

Cooper, R., and Sawaf, A., *Executive E.Q.: Emotional Intelligence in Leadership and Organization* (New York: Perigee Trade, 1998).

Fisher, R., Patton, B., and Ury, W., *Getting to Yes: Negotiating Agreement Without Giving In* (Boston: Houghton Mifflin, 1992).

Jones, R., "Conceptual Development of Nurse-Physician Collaboration," *Holistic Nurse Practice* 8 (3): 1–11 (1994).

Kramer, M., and Schmalenberg, C., "Securing Good Nurse Physician Relationships," *Nursing Management* (July 2003).

Leebov, W., *Assertiveness Skills for Healthcare Professionals* (Lincoln, NE: iUniverse, 2003).

Maurer, R., *Feedback Toolkit: 16 Tools for Better Communication in the Workplace* (New York: Productivity Press, 1994).

Neuhauser, P., *Tribal Warfare in Organizations: Turning Tribal Conflict into Negotiated Peace* (New York: Collins, 1990).

Paterson, R., *The Assertiveness Workbook: How to Express Your Ideas and Stand Up for Yourself at Work and in Relationships* (Oakland, CA: New Harbinger Publications, 2000).

Patterson, K., Grenny, J., McMillan, R., and Switzler, A., *Crucial Conversations: Tools for Talking when Stakes Are High* (New York: McGraw-Hill, 2002).

Reichheld, F., *Loyalty Rules! How Today's Leaders Build Lasting Relationships* (Cambridge, MA: Harvard Business School Press, 2003).

Scott, S., *Fierce Conversations: Achieving Success at Work and in Life One Conversation at a Time* (New York: Berkley Trade, 2004).

Stone, D., Patton, B., Heen, S., and Fisher, R., *Difficult Conversations: How to Discuss What Matters Most* (New York: Penguin, 2000).

## On Enhancing the Patient Experience

Baker, S. K., *Managing Patient Expectations: The Art of Finding and Keeping Loyal Patients* (San Francisco: Jossey-Bass, 1998).

Beeson, S., *Practicing Excellence: A Physician's Manual to Exceptional Health Care* (Gulf Breeze, FL: Fire Starter Publishing, 2006).

Bergeson, S. C., and Dean, J. D., "A Systems Approach to Patient-Centered Care," *Journal of the American Medical Association* 296 (23): 2848–51 (2006).

Berwick, D., Godfrey, A. B., and Roessner, J., *Curing Health Care: New Strategies for Quality Improvement* (San Francisco: Jossey-Bass, 2002).

Berwick, D., Wasson, J. H., et al., "Technology for Patient-Centered, Collaborative Care," *Journal of Ambulatory Care Management* 47 [special issue] (June 22, 2006).

Conway, J., Johnson, B., Edgman-Levitan, S., et al., "Partnering with Patients and Families to Design a Patient- and Family-Centered Health Care System: A Roadmap for the Future," unpublished report from the Institute for Healthcare Improvement, available for free download from www.IHI.org.

Frampton, S., Gilpin, L., and Charmel, P., *Putting Patients First: Designing and Practicing Patient-Centered Care* (San Francisco: Jossey-Bass, 2003).

Gerteis, M., Edgman-Levitan, S., Daley, J., and Delbanco, T., eds., *Through the Patient's Eyes: Understanding and Promoting Patient-Centered Care* (San Francisco: Jossey-Bass, 1993).

Institute for Patient and Family-Centered Care, "Advancing the Practice of Patient- and Family-Centered Care: How to Get Started," unpublished report, available for free download from www.family-centeredcare.org.

Institute for Patient and Family-Centered Care, "Hospitals Moving Forward with Family-Centered Care," unpublished report, available for free download from www.familycenteredcare.org.

Joint Commission, *Patients as Partners: How to Involve Patients and Families in Their Own Care* (Oak Brook Terrace, IL: Joint Commission Resources, 2006).

Lee, F., *If Disney Ran Your Hospital: 9 1/2 Things You Would Do Differently* (Bozeman, MT: Second River Healthcare, 2004).

Leebov, W., Afriat, S., and Presha, J., *Service Savvy Health Care: One Goal at a Time* (Chicago: AHA Press, 1998).

Leebov, W., and Scott, G., *Service Quality Improvement: The Customer Satisfaction Strategy for Health Care* (Lincoln, NE: Authors Choice Press, 2007).

Leebov, W., Scott, G., and Olson, L., *Achieving Impressive Customer Service: Strategies for the Health Care Manager* (Chicago: AHA Press, 1998).

Press, I., *Patient Satisfaction: Understanding and Managing the Experience of Care* (Chicago: Health Administration Press, 2005).

Stubblefield, A., *The Baptist Healthcare Journey to Excellence: Creating a Culture that WOWs!* (New York: John Wiley, 2004).

Studer, Q., *Hardwiring Excellence: Purpose, Worthwhile Work, Making a Difference* (Gulf Breeze, FL: Fire Starter Publishing, 2004).

# Index

*(continued)*